I0460842

Walk in Faith
&
Medicine

Kedrick Pickering M.D.

Walk in Faith & Medicine

Copyright © 2024 by Dr. Kedrick Pickering
All rights reserved.

No part of this publication may be reproduced, distributed, or
transmitted in any form or by any means, including photocopying,
recording, or other electronic or mechanical methods, without the
prior written permission of the publisher, except in the case of brief
quotations embodied in reviews and certain other noncommercial
uses permitted by copyright law. For permission requests, write to
the publisher at info@kedrickpickering.com

This is a work of nonfiction. However, the names, identifying details,
and certain circumstances have been changed to protect the privacy
of individuals. While the author has made every effort to ensure the
accuracy of the information herein, this book is not intended as a
substitute for professional advice. The author and publisher disclaim
any liability arising directly or indirectly from the use or input of this
book.

The views expressed in this book are those of the author and do not
necessarily reflect the views of the publisher or any affiliated
organizations.

ISBN: 979-8-30343-127-0
Second Edition

A FREEDOM MASTERS BOOK

Published by

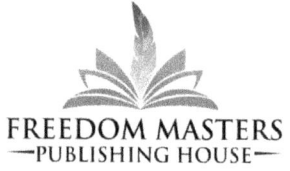

FREEDOM MASTERS
—PUBLISHING HOUSE—

FREEDOM MASTERS PUBLISHING HOUSE LDA

Estr do Castelo 230H
Albufeira, Portugal
8200-385

Walk in Faith
&
Medicine

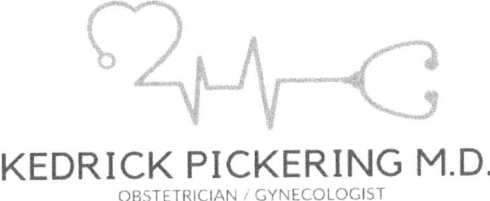

KEDRICK PICKERING M.D.
OBSTETRICIAN / GYNECOLOGIST

www.KedrickPickering.com

Walk In Faith & Medicine

CONTENTS

DEDICATION

"The concept, the mystery of faith, baffles me. This book is dedicated to two persons: First, to you, the reader, whom I wish to inspire with hope. And second, to my patients, from whom I have learned so many of life's lessons.

Working in the field of Obstetrics, Gynaecology and women's health, I have had some very unique and amazing experiences. From being at the birth of many babies, I have seen such joy with their first cry, and I have witnessed the suffering as a mother took her last breath from the debilitating effects of cancer.

I've been able to appreciate the joy and suffering of every step of this journey called life. However, witnessing others' challenges has pushed me to contemplate my own mortality... and still today, I wonder, struggle, and grapple with what the role faith has, in my own life, especially as a physician.

I share here firsthand experiences from which I am of the conviction that there was the presence of an Unseen Hand. I continue to believe so I can understand, and I cry, like the father pleading for help for his dying son: "Lord, I believe; help thou my unbelief" (Mark 9:24). Through my experiences as both a witness and participant, I hope and trust that I inspire you in your daily walk and your journey through life - especially your walk in faith...

ACKNOWLEDGMENTS

The process of writing this book is a book in itself. Laboring to write and the ultimate 'birthing' of this book needed much encouragement over a prolonged period of time. Saying thanks to all who have contributed and have been instrumental, helpful, and critical in this delivery is too simple to show the deep sense of appreciation I feel for you all, but I have to say thanks anyway.

I have been intimidated and scared by the very thought of writing about my personal faith in my professional life. This has taken a lot of courage, and I am eternally grateful to all who have played a role along the way - no matter how great or small it has been.

Family is everything... My dear beloved wife, Alice Marie Henry-Pickering, probably knows the story behind every experience in this book. A nurse/midwife and my partner for over thirty-five years (thirty-one years of marriage), she has been with me through thick and thin in not only my personal life, but on my professional journey as well. Thank you, my dearest.

Our children, all four of them, whom I love dearly - Omonike, Koiya, Khalil, and Kezia are all simply phenomenal and have been very supportive and encouraging. And the little missy - our grandchild Kalei, who has been most inspirational as I write for the future. Thanks to my sister, my brother, all my nieces and nephews, and all my cousins, who have been inspirational in their own ways.

Thanks to the elders in my community where I grew up and still live. Thanks to my late parents and grandparents, who taught me the basic principles of right and wrong and taught

3

me to respect and fear God at an early age.

Thanks to all my teachers from elementary school through high school. It would be difficult and near impossible to write names, for I cannot recall any of my teachers who were discouragers. They all believed in my abilities and encouraged me to strive.

At the University of the West Indies, where I did all of my university education, I did encounter a few who sought to demoralize and discredit me. But to those, I say thank you as well. Your actions and words served as a source of inspiration for me, to prove you wrong.

In medical school and through my residency, Professors Hugh H. Wynter, Joseph Frederick, and Lennox Matadial were mentors and encouragers. To them, I say thanks.

I have been most blessed throughout my entire life to have very close friends who have been there for me no matter the circumstances. I want to say special thanks to Robert, Clyde, and Neil, who all read an initial part of my words on paper and gave invaluable feedback. My friend Bolo, who is a constant inspiration and encourager.

To all my friends from university and classmates from medical school who have encouraged me over the years in one way or another, I say thanks. I have to say a special thank you to my friends and colleagues, Dr. George Mansoor and Dr. Shawn Wynter, for their help and support during medical school and beyond. And thanks to my brethren all in Antigua with whom we have shared a common bond since our early years at university in the seventies - Daven, Brian, Hyram, and Colin.

To my late friend and brother, Everette (Fisher) O'Neal, thanks for the life we shared.

Thanks to all the staff and fellow Laborers at the House of Assembly and the Ministry of Natural Resources and Labor, Government of the British Virgin Islands, for the support while I was there. Special thanks to Mrs. Michelle Bhajan for all the secretarial assistance during those years and beyond.

Thanks to my medical colleagues, the nurses, and all the members of staff at Peebles Hospital and The Dr. D.O. Smith Hospital, where I have worked for nearly forty years. Special thanks to the midwives over the years - Sisters Bertie, Pemberton, Williams, Denny, Barnor, Benjamin, Frett, George, Scotland - and everyone else.

To the staff in the operating room over the years with whom we shared long and tiresome hours: we worked as a team. Thanks. I have to mention Sisters Boyce, Wisdom, Ephraim, and Hoosely - those prayers during difficult moments were invaluable.

There are persons who, along the way, in their own unknown manner, have encouraged me to write. Thanks to Russel Harrigan of Business BVI, Benito Wheatley, Ayana Hull, Angelle Cameron, and Maureen Peters. Thanks to my brothers from our weekly program Body and Soul: Revs Keith Lewis, Michael Anthony, Calvin Mills, and my original cohost, Melvin M. Turnbull. Our journey has been priceless.

Thanks to Dr. Charles Wheatley, Teacher Jeanie Wheatley, Eileen Lucia Parsons, and Dr. Michael O'Neal - the keepers of the records who are constantly encouraging documentation of our life's journeys. Thanks to my friends and companions Dr. Irad and Dr. Marcia Potter - the journey continues.

As I have travelled, my life has intertwined with the following persons in various and unique ways, and in their own ways, they have encouraged the writing process: Olga Samples Davis, Remar Sutton, Dan Buettner, Lisa Nichols, and Ryan Chute. Thank you for the encouragement.

Dr. D. Orlando Smith, my colleague, mentor, and friend since 1986 - the person who has held my hand and been at the side of the operating table in the best of times and the worst - I am simply grateful and say thanks to you. Our journey together, especially when we were alone and had to rely upon each other - is the basis of this book.

This book came together at the time it did, because of a divine meeting at a Lisa Nichols conference in the City of Angels. As fate would have it, Carrie Kohan and I sat next to each other on the first morning. We chatted a bit during the session and continued to interact throughout the 3-day event. "You should hire me to help you write that book," were her words. The rest is history... Carrie, you have been a coach extraordinaire, and this book is a result of your skills and dedication to helping me get it done in the time we originally set forth. Structure is what I was looking for, and you gave it, along with your guidance and encouragement - especially in those first sessions... you've been invaluable. Thanks.

To write a book about faith means that there is an object of that faith. Thank you to God Almighty, through His son Jesus Christ, who loves even me. That He loves me continues to boggle my mind. As I journey and grow, and my faith deepens... I believe in the power of God to move mountains.

To understand the love of God for a wretched soul like me is mystifying, and I can only say how eternally grateful I am that He extends His love toward me. Thank you God, from whom all blessings flow, for giving me the strength and courage to complete this task.

Introduction

"Are you sure you are going to be okay? " my wife asked me as she was being wheeled into the operating room, I was the surgeon who was about to perform an emergency Caesarean Section on my beloved spouse... Not by choice of course, but because I was the only practicing Obstetrician at the time in our small Caribbean community hospital.

"You can't have faith and don't have faith," was my response to her. There wasn't the time or the luxury to even think about any emotional involvement; we had to proceed and trust that everything would be alright.

This was one of many examples during my years of practice where I grappled with the subject of faith and the mystery of it all. I have wrestled continually with the biblical imperative: "To seek God first, and all other things you want will seek after you." How do I do that in a world where everyday living calls for work, mortgage payments, childcare, and growing bills in the hustle and bustle to enjoy the "good life"?

I am a medical doctor, trained to take care of others, not necessarily myself. And as I continue to help others, I've come to realize I need to care for myself or

I shall perish as well, sooner than later. This is why I began to write; It is my release...

And so, the birthing of my book began. I let go of the limiting beliefs I had. Many of these beliefs had been indoctrinated into me during the years of medical training and the pressures of being 'the only one' on the island where my family and I lived. I had a belief that I could never say no, and I still believe that to a certain extent. But what I have learned is that I also have to say 'Yes' to myself, as well as to my family. Society has put many professions on pedestals, forgetting that the people in those industries are as frail as the next human being. The only difference is that in my profession, we wear a white coat and carry a stethoscope. Our human nature, our needs and wants, are not negated by status.

Like many, I've had to work under some extremely challenging situations. Only in my case, as an Obstetrician/Gynaecologist, every day was about birth or death... Dealing with stillbirths when there were no warning signs (in an otherwise normal pregnancy) were some of the worst experiences for everyone concerned – including all the hospital staff. We all felt the loss, from the head nurse to the receptionists and cleaning staff. We were all a team, and the dilemma I faced with such immense grief and no direct support system (in a pre-internet era) was heart-wrenching! I found I was constantly questioning myself, "What did we do wrong? What else should we have done?"

But the real question for not only myself, but our entire team was, "Where and who do we turn to for help with our own emotional trauma, now that the immediate storm has passed?'' It is the sequel to this that lingers and is the most painful.

The limited medical staff that we had in our hospital also suffered equally, if not worse, with their own pain and feelings of loss, As the surgeon in charge, like the conductor directing the orchestra, all eyes were on me. I didn't have the time to grieve like the others, but the need was no less intense. Sometimes, I'd cry in my subconscious mind and hope and believe that the voice within me heard my sorrow loud and clear. Like a child crying to their parents, needing relief from their suffering, I did the same by relying on the Almighty - waiting for Him to respond.

Being in the operating room in the wee hours of the morning, when all medical knowledge and facilities were failing us - we needed help. And where our beliefs in our abilities were weakening, I'd find myself pleading for the Divine to intervene. Inevitably, just when all felt lost, a sense of peace would wash over the operating room. Our entire team would become calm, and in the silence, a peaceful presence would come, in the midst of these storms. It seemed that every time we would turn to prayer, the Unseen Hand would show up. It is most difficult to explain, but we all felt it... And the outcomes were more than what we could ever have imagined.

During these moments of 'do or die' was where I have come closest to understanding faith. I am told that faith happens when there is a concern... and in these most delicate of situations, reliance on the Almighty is all you have left.

I have been familiar with family and patients alike saying to me, "Doctor, we'll be praying for you and the staff," especially before major surgery. It is a bit unusual, however, if I dare say uncomfortable, when someone says at the patient's bedside, "Let us pray together." Doctors are supposed to be in charge, not delegate that authority to someone else. And certainly not push their faith upon another who may have differing beliefs. But I found myself in this very instance, when a patient who was extremely ill asked me to pray with them. She needed surgical intervention and was in a precarious state. The miraculous recovery after prolonged surgery, in the very face of what appeared to be advanced cancer, could only have been attributed to those prayers and divine help.

These are the kinds of experiences of faith and medicine I share with you in this book. They are all real stories, but the names and times are amended to maintain privacy. The experiences are as they occurred, with the underlying theme of how faith played an integral role in the conclusion of each event. They were all clinical situations. More often than not, life or death in nature...

Nothing can prepare you for these events, especially given that I grew up in a small village on an island in the Caribbean during a time when technology was a distant dream. In my formative years, modern facilities were far from the order of the day. Running water, electricity, flushing toilets, and telephones were all utilities that evolved in my community while I was growing up. I only knew one person in my childhood years who had gone away and become a doctor. Radio was the predominant and common means of communication. Everything outside of the village seemed eons away. There wasn't much to dream about... I had no real reason to think of becoming anything else outside of my village.

We were taught that there was a Deity, a Supreme Being beyond and before us. If we were good boys and girls, Creator would be nice to us... But if we were naughty, we'd be spanked by an angry God. I personally feared God as a youth because of this. Not much was imparted about a loving, caring, forgiving God - and concepts like faith were too complex I guess, for a young villager such as myself.

The one thing that stayed with me was that our elders believed in the Divine for a better life, and they prayed and believed daily.

This book is not a theological transcript, nor is it a religious theoretical prescription of any kind. It is also not a premise for some church doctrine. I have no training or qualifications in these areas. It is not a book of success stories; in fact, there are some heart-wrenching and heartbreaking stories where failure was outright painful. The lessons of compassion, forgiveness, faith, and moving forward in unconditional love, have been the most welcomed outcomes.

Many of these events I share with you here, happened during a period in my early professional life - when I worked alone as the only Obstetrics and Gynaecology in our community hospital.

As I've said earlier, all of these stories are real – but in writing and compiling these events, I had an unexpected outcome in writing this book... Just as the inner voice prescribed the remedy of putting my stories to paper... it has given me relief from some of the most trying and traumatic moments of my life. To the point that I now ask myself in wonder, "How did we make it through all of these adrenaline-pumping moments in time?"

My movement forward in 'Doctor Heal Thyself' began as an overwhelming urge to put my thoughts on paper. An internal nudge that haunted me for some time. This pressing feeling began as a series of questions that seemed to be answered by a voice within. As I'd frantically asked myself, ''Where do I find time to care for myself? My schedule is at its limit already!'' I found myself hearing wise, compassionate words within me say, ''Trust the space will open for your healing, if you desire it to do so''. I then asked, ''And where do I find the resources to invest in seeking the Divine? I'm spent energetically already. I have no energy left for myself or my pursuit of faith.'' The Inner Voice quickly replied with, ''Strength and fortitude will be given to those who seeketh.'' I protested and said in frustration, ''But what if I've reached the end of my human abilities?'' There was silence, and then I heard the compassionate voice within say, ''Start with the first step... Lift your pen and write. Release all that is within you and help others in the process."

I'd like to share with you a final thought that this is not a book that speaks strictly about Miracles, even though I have witnessed two miracles during my professional career. (These true miracles were separate and apart from the many instances of miraculous recoveries, where I have marveled at the outcomes). Instead, this book is more about the fact that while I admit that our team's work was always within the medical protocol, I have to conclude that there was also an extra unseen hand guiding us as we prayed for divine intervention during those seconds, minutes, and hours of saving our patient's life.

This book does tell you the stories I've experienced without trying to explain the outcomes. I have presented the evidence as I have gone through the trials and tribulations that ensued. And I've come to believe that…

'Faith has to work for it to work… and as I have seen it, I have shared it'. The verdict is now yours to contemplate.'

As Ralph Waldo Emerson once said:

"Life is a journey, not a destination."

So, thank you for joining me on this journey and may these stories inspire an inner dialogue that guides you in your own life's pursuits. I trust you will find the beauty in the mundane and the faith within to carry you forward.

No chance at all if you think you can pull it off by yourself. Every chance in the world if you trust God to do it.
Matthew 19:26

JOURNAL 1

MIRACLE

There was an odd calm and peaceful reassurance in the delivery room that morning despite the baby being born unresponsive. It was a normal labor, with the usual ups and downs… the ebb and flow of moments filled with pain, pushing, and persistence leading to delivery. The parents were mature; the mother was multiparous (multiple pregnancies) and had already indicated that this was her last child. She wanted no more pregnancies, even though both parents were very excited about the birth of this baby.

Nothing during the labor could have prepared us for what looked like a disastrous outcome. The baby was born ashen grey. Her tongue was protruding from the mouth, and she was 'flat' with no body tone. In medical jargon, the baby was born blue, with no signs of life. We immediately recognised that the umbilical cord was wrapped around the neck three times. We could not detect a heartbeat, and the electronic fetal heart rate monitoring device gave no warning signs as to this outcome, during the labor. In other words, we did not see this coming...

The parents were fully aware that something was wrong. The baby did not cry, and anxiety began to build in the room. The mother, clinging to her husband out of desperation. She cried out, "Oh my God, what's wrong with my baby?" Against that background, we glanced at each other without allowing our own anxieties to show. Automatic responses took over. We knew the clock was ticking, and we were in a race against time to save this baby's life.

The process of resuscitation began immediately once the cord was cut, and the baby was separated from the mother.

There were three of us in the delivery room - two nurse midwives and me - each taking our roles as per established protocols for such emergencies. We were taught the basics of management in resuscitation, and these were carried out without a hiccup. Despite our experience, we were worried because this was obviously a life-and-death situation. Yet, we executed our protocols efficiently.

Seconds into such a crisis can seem like an eternity. We were sweating in the air-conditioned room. It felt like our heart rates were pounding loud enough to hear above the echoes of the machines. The parents stared at us, exasperated with worry. The need for help pushed us to reach beyond ourselves, avoiding the grip of fear.

I have made it a habit to say a quiet prayer asking for divine intervention in such cases, and this was no exception. The mother's background crying turned into weeping and howling as the seconds ticked by. When the odds are stacked against us professionally, we become painfully aware of the limits of our knowledge and expertise. A measure of faith becomes extremely reassuring. Over the years, witnessing successful outcomes has bolstered my confidence in the presence of the Almighty. We performed our duties. We were frantic but diligent - looking for hopeful signs as we waited for divine intervention.

Resuscitation efforts yielded hope within the first few minutes as a heartbeat was detected. The pediatrician was called, but as is often the case in our small community hospital, the pediatrician was not readily available and had to be summoned from afar. Several minutes went by, which seemed like an eternity. Despite our anxiety, we persisted with the resuscitation, ensuring a good oxygen supply for this little one.

The baby remained flat, but we were encouraged when we noted the pink color of her lips - a hopeful sign that oxygen was being supplied. Throughout the resuscitation, we had completely ignored the mother except for occasional glances to check for any signs of excessive bleeding.

We were relieved when the pediatrician arrived. He quickly took over, intubating the baby. He established an intravenous line and prepared her for transfer to the neonatal intensive care unit down the hallway.

Our attention turned back to the mother. Luckily, there was no excessive bleeding, though the placenta was still undelivered. As the placenta was delivered, we continued praying for a miracle. The father, though composed, remained deeply concerned while the mother bombarded us with repeated questions: "Doc, is my baby going to be okay? Will she survive? What should we expect?"

We had to complete the mother's post-delivery care despite being as uncertain as she was about the baby's future. Transferring the mother to a more comfortable room, we assured her that we needed to wait for the pediatrician's updates.

Finally, I made it to the intensive care unit for an update. The first indication of a miracle was seeing a pink, living baby. She was attached to tubes and lines and was assisted by a ventilator. The room was calm, machines beeping steadily as the neonatal team worked efficiently. There was hope in the air, and the uplifting atmosphere was inspiring.

Encouraged, I returned to the parents, reporting that the baby was alive and showing signs of improvement. The medical team's smiles throughout the room further reassured us.

As minutes turned to hours, the baby's condition stabilized. The intensity of team persisted, but signs of improvement uplifted our spirits. The parents visited regularly, staying by the incubator while being comforted by the staff. The mother was discharged 36 hours later, with full privileges to visit the baby as needed.

The recovery was miraculously sustained with no setbacks. Medical chatter was continually optimistic, and the calm reassurance lingered. Seven days later, the baby was discharged to her home without treatment. Regular follow-ups showed normal neuro-developmental milestones, and the parents' gratitude was immensely rewarding.

Some might attribute this outcome to our medical skills and timely interventions. While these were critical, it is hard to ignore the peace and calm that surrounded us in those urgent moments.

There is nothing more devastating in obstetrics than a stillbirth or maternal death, each profoundly affecting the parents, family members, and medical staff. Sometimes though, we are surprised by the Unseen Hand that guides our thoughts and actions, and shows us life, where once there was none.

This particular intervention continues to make me reflect on the role of prayer in medicine. It lingers in my mind, occupying some of my deepest thoughts, as I navigate the challenges of my professional life.

Life is what you make it, but it won't happen on its own – Kedrick Pickering

JOURNAL 2

BECOMING A DOCTOR

Fifty years ago, dreaming of becoming a doctor felt as unreachable as travelling to another Universe might seem today. Growing up on a small island, life was shaped by the absence of electricity, running water, and telephones, with no mass media to broaden our horizons. Our only connection to the outside world was a small transistor radio that served the entire community. In those days, the idea of someone from my background becoming a medical doctor was almost mythical - more like a fairy tale than a reality. I knew of only one local figure... a dentist who had achieved such a feat, and even he seemed like a legend rather than a real person.

Fast forward to today, and one of my offspring holds a postgraduate degree in forensic science and is preparing to advance further into cybersecurity. The difference between our worlds, just two generations apart, could not be more striking. Yet, my own journey to becoming a physician likely began during those same high school years, sparked by an unexpected conversation with one of my most inspiring teachers.

Mr, Yamraj, my geology and geography teacher, was a man of vision. He had been recruited from Guyana as part of an initiative to strengthen our developing education system. We had too few trained local teachers and educators... So, professionals from other Caribbean nations came to fill the gaps, and they brought with them a wealth of knowledge and fresh perspectives.

One day in high school, Mr. Yamraj approached and casually asked me what I planned to do after graduation. Perhaps my youthful naivety or my lack of ambition frustrated him. I replied that I planned to study rocks, retreat to the hills, and live as a hermit.

His response was both fiery and transformative: "Boy Kedrick, don't talk foolishness!" he bolstered! "You should get a scholarship, go abroad, and study to become a doctor. Then come back and help your country" he added.

That moment felt like a bolt of lightning! Both chastisement and inspiration wrapped into one! It planted a seed however. One that grew alongside the values instilled in me by my parents, my community, and my faith.

My mother, in particular, was instrumental in shaping my intellectual curiosity. She nurtured my love for reading from an early age... seeking out whatever books and materials she could find (even in the resource-scarce 1960s).

Her encouragement was unwavering, and her belief in my potential helped me to see a future beyond the limitations of our small island. Even now, reading remains one of my greatest joys. A habit that has served me well in both life and medicine.

Faith also played a profound role in my development. Both Church and Sunday school were cornerstones of our community, shaping not only our spiritual lives but also our social interactions, and sense of purpose. These early experiences taught me about ambition, service, and the importance of building a better community. However, my relationship with God was complex.

As a child, I viewed Creator like He was both distant and demanding, a figure quick to judge and punish. But over time my faith deepened - shaped by my experiences as a physician. I came to see God as a source of compassion, guidance, and love. A perspective that has undoubtedly made me a better doctor.

One memory stands out vividly from my childhood: a book left at our home by visiting missionaries. The book was filled with pictures of people helping others in far-off lands. This left an indelible impression on me. It wasn't just the images that stayed with me - it was the idea that caring for others could be a calling. In those moments, perhaps without even realizing it, I began to dream of a life centered on compassion and service.

Today as a physician, I remain deeply attuned to the social circumstances of my patients. I understand, perhaps more than most, how the smallest seeds of encouragement, faith, and opportunity can grow into something extraordinary. Reflecting on my journey, I can see how these early influences like my teacher's words, my mother's sacrifices, or the missionaries' book, have shaped not only my career, but also my commitment to making a difference in this corner of the planet.

Dreams take many forms, and our lives are shaped by a constellation of influences. Looking back, I marvel at how each seemingly small moment played a role in leading me and my family, to where we are today.

"Faith is taking the first step even when you don't see
the whole staircase"
Martin Luther King Jr

JOURNAL 3

WORST NIGHTMARE

There were pivotal moments in my career when I realized that the practice of medicine alone wasn't enough - belief in a sustaining power was needed. During medical school, the Professor of Pediatrics taught us that we must always take the death of a child seriously, no matter the cause. However, no one prepares you for how devastating it is to deliver and hold a stillborn baby... especially when you feel accountable and answerable to everyone involved.

Delivering a dead baby is absolutely devastating! Holding a lifeless body in your hands is profoundly heavy. One immediate question enters your mind, "What went wrong?" Then, a flood of emotions and a stream of unanswered questions follow - as was the case with this couple who came into the hospital on this most difficult of days.

This was their first pregnancy - a time filled with excitement, joy, and anticipation. From their first prenatal visit to their last, it had been a wonderful experience. Each milestone was celebrated, from the confirmation of pregnancy to the first ultrasound, hearing the heartbeat for the first time, and everything in between. I tell all my patients on hearing that first heartbeat, "That is the sweetest sound you will hear until you hear your baby cry." Together we build excitement, looking forward as all of our anticipation grew.

As the pregnancy progressed, all lab tests were normal, all maternal parameters were in order, and everything was moving along smoothly. I reassured them that we were expecting a normal delivery - all signs pointed in that direction. They attended Lamaze classes at the right time and even visited the maternity ward to orient themselves. They were as well-prepared for labor as any couple could be... patiently waiting for the appointed hour. In my approach to pregnancy care, I emphasize to all our patients, to be patient and take one step at a time - no matter their excitement. While we are in an anticipatory place, I try to remind them you can't take home a baby until the baby is born. So, we take one day at a time.

Labor started normally, right around the expected date. All admitting protocols to the maternity ward were followed. The labor progressed without concern; she needed minimal analgesia, and delivery was imminent. The moments of painful contractions were interspersed by the expectant joy ahead.

Her attending midwife stayed with her for the entire duration, despite her shift being over. The patient handled labor and delivery well, clearly benefitting from the Lamaze classes. And her husband did a fantastic job encouraging her. Maternal vital signs and fetal heart rate remained normal throughout. Everyone in the delivery room was actively engaged, as we usually are, with encouragement to push and push a little harder. She gave it her all, and with the final two contractions, she was able to push the head out without any tearing or laceration.

The baby was delivered without difficulty and looked perfectly normal - but it didn't cry. The umbilical cord was cut, and the baby was transferred to the resuscitation table, where all protocols were followed... but there was no heartbeat. The baby didn't take a breath. No cry, and all resuscitation attempts failed. The mood in the delivery room was dark and somber. You could hear each other's breathing with the depth of despair that had entered the room. The reality of the moment caved in on us like a brick wall.

The mother's wailing erupted and could probably be heard around the world. Every one of us in that delivery room was in total shock and disbelief. "How could this happen? What went so terribly wrong? What else could we have done? Is this a nightmare? This can't be real."

The room was filled with tears, distress, and a mountain of emotional despair. Thirty years later while writing this, it is as if I've stepped back in time and can see and feel the level of sorrow all over again. It is as if I'm reliving those moments - despite the wide range of emotional challenges I've encountered since -

during my long career. Not a second is forgotten! I remember it all.

There were no warning signs; we had just experienced a brand-new stillbirth... what a devastating blow to the parents, family, and hospital staff. As the one in charge of the OR, a loss such as this carries an even greater burden on your heart. One that is difficult to explain.

As traumatic as the event was, it was made even worse with the mother's devastation and nonstop cries... for nearly twenty-four hours she howled in agony! She was inconsolable to the point of near mental and physical exhaustion. The husband's pain was magnified by his inability to comfort his wife, and our sadness grew with them both.

At the time, we didn't have a professional crisis management team or full-time psychiatric or psychological counselling to help with grief. The patient, against our advice (and understandably so), asked to be discharged the next day. She couldn't bear the sounds of babies crying in the ward.

I had dealt with stillbirths before, but none as harrowing as this. This was unbearably tough for all concerned. We cared for the patient and family members, yet in those days, there was no one to care for us, the first responders and hospital staff. We'd go home alone and listen to the echos of that mother's anguish in our minds for days, weeks or even years.

This aspect of grief is often overlooked. We had no answers for the stillbirth, but to face a barrage of questions - from both ourselves and others. Amid the suffering was the guilt we felt. The constant replay of the event in our minds... What did we do wrong? What could we have done differently? Was this our fault or was it simply unavoidable?

The range of questions is mind-boggling, yet you still have to put on a brave face and pretend all is well. The daily tasks must go on, work continues, babies are still being born, and shattered confidence cannot interfere with your performance. Patients in the ward knew about the incident and needed reassurance that it wouldn't happen to them. As the only obstetrician at the time, all eyes were on me...

Life in a small community has its positives and negatives, and in this moment - I questioned where to find the strength and courage to continue on. How do you prevent fear from creeping into your daily work and shattering your confidence?

This was not a sprint; the grief and reactions to grief can last a very long time without counselling. And after four to six months - prolonged grief can become pathological. In extreme cases, an autopsy might have provided answers, but unfortunately, it wasn't readily available. We could have sought assistance from an overseas pathologist. However, the patient was strongly opposed to this. So, with no outside help, we had to support the parents through every stage, including funeral arrangements. The medical team directly involved attended the funeral, not only as a means of support for the family, but also to help in our own grieving. Closure was nowhere in sight.

Close friends, who were professionals and had faced a neonatal death themselves years earlier, offered tremendous support and even served as surrogate counsellors. This was a relief, as they helped carry the emotional burden. The two mothers formed a bond, and the support was invaluable. Yet, the patient's grief became pathological; she developed severe postpartum depression.

Our facility didn't have the resources to treat this, and she was referred overseas. I saw them regularly, every six to eight weeks, and although she was receiving expert care at a specialized facility, her recovery was slow.

She was relentless in her search for answers about her baby's death and joined a support group she found during her travels.

Watching her journey through grief was incredibly tough, I had nothing left in my reserves, and even my words of encouragement faded with time - becoming almost rhetorical. But the staff and I had to keep going. Each visit with her reopened those memories of the delivery room. We all had to find the strength to move forward and not let this painful experience define us as professionals. Oh Physician, heal thyself.

There was a unique aspect to this experience, working in a small community hospital in the early nineties. There was no internet, and long-distance calls were prohibitively expensive. Finding help and support was nearly impossible. So, fast forward to today, where technology allows constant interactions and consultations with colleagues just a WhatsApp message away... Thirty-plus years ago, that wasn't even a dream.

Today, our same hospital has various services and several other obstetrics colleagues. A stillbirth now prompts natural support and solidarity among the team. This spontaneous camaraderie means no one bears the emotional burden alone. Such a support system would have been invaluable back then, but it simply didn't exist.

I remember waking up in a hotel room in Europe during a business trip in the middle of the night a few years ago. The room was pitch black; I was disoriented. Trying to find the bathroom, I was utterly lost. I had no sense of direction and none to turn to. It was a moment of despair until I managed to turn on a light.

Navigating the trauma of that stillbirth felt much like that experience in that dark hotel room. I needed a light to guide me, to learn to trust in that light by first believing it existed. Step by step, I learned to climb a staircase I couldn't see. Each day I made it through without added guilt, felt like a small victory... allowing me to trust in the Unseen Hand. It didn't always feel real, but it was reassuring and made the journey less daunting. I couldn't imagine what the family were going through! But personally, I had to continually search for Divine help and guidance for a prolonged period of time to prevent that particular experience from derailing me professionally.
St. John the Divine wrote,

"Experience isn't what happens to a man. It is what a man does with what happens to him."

Each step of this journey has challenged my thinking and strengthened my belief in the role of faith, and I continue to marvel how work manifests faith.

"God moves in a mysterious way, His wonders to perform"
William Cowper

JOURNAL 4

DIGNITY

Mr. Cline was an elderly gentleman when I first met him. Our encounter took place at a public health clinic where I worked during my internship in the mid-eighties. He had lived abroad and experienced the world wars. He was a proud, dignified man who was suffering from a chronic leg ulcer. His only living relative, as far as I was aware, was a niece and her extended family, who were his caregivers.

Our encounter in the clinic came about because he was seeking care for his leg ulcer and other medical ailments associated with aging. He was in his mid-eighties when we met, and he subsequently became a regular at the clinic where I worked. He was transported to and from the clinic by his niece. Occasionally, he would mix up his appointments and attend on a day when I wasn't there. Yet, he would simply sit and wait until I was available.

He never complained. He would tell the nurse or whoever was working, "Just inform Dr. Pickering that I'm waiting." He obviously appreciated the care extended to him and was most grateful every time. He was always prepared to wait patiently and never murmured a word of discontent.

We developed a bond of friendship and mutual respect. I've always held great respect for the older generations, probably due in part to the time I spent with my grandfather during my teenage years and the relationship I had with my parents. Mr. Cline had to attend the clinic regularly, and it became very taxing on his family, particularly his niece.

After realizing the strain on his family from bringing him to the clinic (sometimes weekly), I volunteered to do home care for him without any financial remuneration. I had grown to love and respect him as if he were family and wanted to do my best to help him. This gesture, I think, was greatly appreciated by him and his family and brought me immense joy to feel that appreciation.

I worked in that clinic setting for about two years before returning to the university hospital at my alma mater to pursue a residency in Obstetrics and Gynaecology. During my vacation trips home, a visit to Mr. Cline was always in order. I remember on how two such visits, I arrived at his home unannounced and there he was, sitting in his regular chair, head bowed, either sleeping or praying. With a gentle tap on his shoulder, his eyes would open wide, and the most radiant smile would spread across his face.

"Dr. Pickering!" he would exclaim, with his voice filled with joy, "I was praying for you. I knew you would come." It was always a wonder to me. He always seemed so peaceful and full of positive energy. At the end of each visit, he would pray for me with the most encouraging words, which penetrated my very being. He always ended with,

"I am always praying for you."

My daily journey through life is filled with reminders of those encounters.

Mr. Cline was still alive and well when I completed my residency and returned home permanently. On my first visit with him after earning my qualifications. I informed him of my new skill sets and explained the work I would now be doing. There was a pregnant pause before he responded - I thought he might have fallen asleep. Then he lifted his head, looked me squarely in the eyes and with a heavy, raspy voice (reminiscent of Marlon Brando in *The Godfather*), he'd say, "Dr. Pickering - please remember this: you never put that knife to cut anyone before you pray."

His words were powerful and penetrated deeply. I wear them like a tattoo on my chest and carry them in my heart. I hear his words regularly - practically every time I'm in the operating room.

There have been moments, caught up in the anxiety of the situation, when I've forgotten to pray. But when I realize this, I pause quietly, just to acknowledge the power that comes through prayer, and I offer one. For

Mr. Cline added an important addendum to his advice: "When others see you progressing and being successful, you must know and acknowledge the power of God that is guiding you through your faith and prayers."

These words have been a constant companion, especially during difficult days and nights. There is a sense of an unseen hand, a reassurance that's hard to explain.

In my daily work, Mr. Cline's words have kept me focused on the greater good of what we do. I remain amazed by outcomes in difficult pregnancies where our skills seemed insufficient to justify the results. Living a purposeful and meaningful life is often rooted in such experiences. The birth of a baby and the beauty of a newborn, gives us hope and confidence in the greater sense and meaning of life.

The joy of new parents leaves me yearning to understand and appreciate why we were created. What can we do to recreate that joy and beauty in people's everyday lives?

"Faith and prayer are the vitamins of the soul-man cannot live in health without them" - Mahalia Jackson

JOURNAL 5

TRUSTING CONSCIENCE

I am a frail vessel trodding along as a human being, only getting by - by the grace that has been extended to me through love and support. I ponder my own mortality on a regular basis and try to make use of the time allotted here on earth. I come face to face with persons having to make life-altering decisions almost daily. In my professional work, nothing has given me more pause and cause for deep personal reflection than a patient seeking services for the termination of a pregnancy.

Even though I do not provide such services, people consult me for advice with regards to their decision-making and how to access those services on a regular basis. My struggle is a daily one, a real one, not a figment of my imagination... How can I help without being judgmental and/or condemning? And how can I help within the context of the forces that have shaped my life?

My upbringing taught me to respect the views and sentiments of others, certainly their challenges and suffering. My formative environment is rooted in the rights and wrongs as taught by my elders and the role the church played in those teachings. And then, there is the guiding directive of the Hippocratic Oath that I am bound to take seriously... it was hammered into my psyche throughout my academic career.

I am conflicted, I am a flawed human being with probably more personal faults than any patient I encounter. Who am I to condemn or judge? Every single experience of a patient seeking a termination of pregnancy arouses my consciousness; I listen, counsel, recommend and often refer. Each individual needs and requires nothing more than respect... a listening ear and compassionate heart.

Every time I am confronted with someone seeking termination of a pregnancy, I have to ask myself, "Suppose it was me in a difficult situation needing help and advice? What would I expect from the professional I was seeking help from? Am I doing unto others what I would want them to do to (or for) me?" I find solace and comfort in the words of Paul; "It is not what a man does that determines whether his work is spiritual or temporal; it is why he does it" (Colossians 3:23).

I am a Medical Officer because I want more than anything, to heal, to restore health, to save a life. That is precisely why the realities of my patients and persons who have been referred to me weigh heavily on me and on my spirit, It opens me, more often than not, to listen to that little voice that may alert me as to whether I am doing the right thing for the patient, for humanity, for me.

As I recount some cases, you would recognize the struggles, the realities, the conflicts, and the brushes with the law, as it currently stands in my country. The following stories illustrate some of the real-time dilemmas I have had to deal with.

Mrs A was a married woman in her mid-forties. She had a stable family with three teenage children. She had a bilateral tubal ligation after her last pregnancy twelve years prior. She and her family had migrated from their homeland and had settled into a comfortable living in their new homeland for about seven years.

Upon arriving to my office, it was apparent they were both very nervous individuals. Mrs. A and her husband were the first clients for the day. They had shown up rather early and could hardly wait to speak with me. The air was tense, and I could sense there was some bad news about to be uttered by them both. I did my best to welcome them professionally, as I asked them to have a seat. They both quietly took a seat and looked at me in silence. A nervous smile came across their faces, and before I could offer any words to initiate the dialogue, they both let out a deep sigh, and Mrs A began to speak.

She offered an apology, and said, "Dr P. we are sorry to bother you, but this is as much a burden for us as it will likely be for you." Perplexed, I responded, "Ok... how can I help?" while putting on my best composure to suggest, I was ready to help in any way I could. But under my white lab coat, I could feel my heart beating fast! It was reminiscent of being in a final clinical exam, where the professors were hovering over me – waiting for the correct answer... I took a few deep breaths, and we began.

Mrs. A gathered her composure, but she soon dropped her head and could not speak. It was obvious she was having difficulties finding where to start. Her husband leaned on her shoulder while putting his arm affectionately around her - giving the best emotional support he could offer his wife. Finally, Mrs. A raised her head and began to share that she was extremely concerned because she missed her monthly period. She added she was always regular and that initially she wasn't concerned because she was entering the change of life or menopausal years... but then she started to experience what she described as, 'the unpleasant signs of well... pregnancy!'

Mrs A added that she had a near-death experience during her labour and delivery in her last pregnancy. She had been explicitly warned by her then medical team, that under no circumstances should she become pregnant again! The tubal ligation was done at that time to prevent it from happening again. Although they could not give the exact medical details, it sounded like she had seizures followed by eventual heart failure, ending in intensive care for a few weeks after her delivery.

As I listened to them recount the story, my own nervousness increased, reliving the moments as if I had been the attending physician during that time...

The consultation lasted about an hour, eventually reaching a crescendo. I had to give advice... These were two people of faith who appreciated the complex nature of the dilemma and decision they were facing. The risk of carrying a pregnancy with almost certain death, versus, terminating the pregnancy with personal conflicts in their faith and beliefs.

I of course, could not possibly give information contrary to the previous medical advice that was given in the context of the clinical experience. And I certainly could not give advice against my own conscience either, but the realities were clear. I reinforced the previous medical advice given. They eventually terminated the pregnancy after seeking a second opinion.

I have a professional responsibility which includes referring a patient to another physician for care that is outside my skill sets. For example, someone with a fracture will be referred to an Orthopedic Surgeon. Similarly, for any other speciality, a referral is necessary without imposing any prejudice or personal beliefs - no matter how strong those might be on a personal level.

The obligation is first to do no harm and to provide non-prejudicial care. Lifestyles and their consequences are an existential reality of our human existence, and I was taught to render care to the best of my ability. I spend an inordinate amount of time daily trying to educate and encourage others about their overall health, weight loss, diet and exercise. It is very appealing to be condemning and critical when lifestyles are destructive, especially when poor daily choices are made… but the obligation to be non-judgmental stares me straight in the face. Who am I to judge after all? My role is to help, not hurt, nor harm.

There is one thing alone that stands the brunt of life through its length: A quiet conscience, as recorded in the writings of St John The Divine (1st John 3:21). I have to constantly reflect on the writings of Paul as recorded in the Holy Scriptures. "Oh, wretched man that I am..." What a miserable state I find myself in as I wonder about the end of my days."

I have to constantly ask myself each time, did I do the right thing? Is my conscience clear? I reflect on the personal struggles of King David of biblical times, and I reassure myself that;

"The Lord doesn't see things the way you see them. People judge by outward appearance, but the Lord looks at the heart." (1 Samuel 16:7).

This is not a philosophical or theological battle. This is a deeply personal war raging in my mind every single time I'm faced with what I see as moral decisions. "Am I doing what is right? Is my Creator pleased with me? Can I live with myself in all that I do?" Well, I had many more experiences to test my compass, including Miss T.

Miss T was a single unmarried mother of two. She was in a troubled, unstable relationship. I met her partner during my early years of practice. There was instability

Walk In Faith & Medicine

on all fronts and her family were not fond of her spouse at all. He was the father of several children and was not very supportive. He had been in trouble with the law, and oftentimes, she found herself without basic supplies and needing both emotional and financial support.

In her day-to-day struggles, she found herself leaning on someone she met and ended up in a clandestine affair with him. He offered what she needed most, and she accepted. But despite being on contraception, she found herself pregnant. The guilt was overwhelming for her. She blamed herself, thinking that she was being punished.

Even though he was a married man, he accompanied Miss T to the consultation. Miss T's spouse was quick to request the pregnancy be terminated, She was ambivalent and was resistant to the idea. But, during our conversation she entered into a period of indecision, which created disharmony between them both. The argument began and it became apparent that Miss T was quite attached to her spouse. She wanted to have the baby, yet none of this was known to him.

She visited me twice on her own after the initial consultation, seeking guidance and comfort in her confused and difficult times. There was no easy answer or solution. Ultimately, she had to live with the consequences of whatever decision she would make. It seemed to be an awfully lonely journey for her, and I felt great empathy for her as I tried to help. I did my best Pontius Pilate imitation, while dancing between the decisions to be made. I was confident in my own thoughts based on her circumstances – but ultimately it was their decision.

I did my best job trying to show her the pros and cons of her options, avoiding the path of specifically directing her on what to do. There were times when my empathy towards her was such that I actually felt sorry for her situation. She trusted and valued my input, but I couldn't advise her specifically on what to do. I think she eventually terminated the pregnancy as she didn't return for a follow-up.

I had my share of consultations during the pandemic of persons seeking termination of pregnancies It was a varied and mixed bag; all were life experiences of one form or another.

I live and work next door to the United States Virgin Islands, where before and during the pandemic, termination of pregnancy services was freely available and accessible. Referral across the pond was an uncomplicated process once travel for the individual was permitted. Although with a heavy heart and sometimes a muddied conscience, I honored my professional responsibility and referred persons who consulted me seeking services I do not render.

One consultation that stands out was that of a single, unmarried woman with no entanglements, no children, and a professional in her own right. The pandemic was a lonely, isolated time. Companionship was a desirous commodity. The patient had a friend with no romantic interest, but he provided conversations and a means of regular contact. These conversations eventually led to physical intimacy.

By her account, one of the unintended results of her becoming pregnant, was that she hated the very idea of having a baby at that stage of her life. She didn't even like the person who was the father...and she wanted no part in having a life-long connection with him. In her words, there was no way on earth she was carrying and or having a child with him.

She was well aware I didn't provide services to terminate - all she wanted was for me to guide her in the direction she should go. This was new to her, and these were extraordinary times. She was resolute in her decision and was the least interested in me being compassionate... Although, I certainly did my best to be non-judgmental and help.

During our conversation, I began to wonder what my role was here - given I could only be an ear to hear her concerns. Was my job complete here? Was my conscience clear, or was I an unwilling participant and therefore culpable? I'm still unsure today.

These three cases are examples of real issues I came face to face with, in my daily work. I am aware that 'faith and conscience are a formidable twosome' and my personal struggles are intimately tied to the two. I use my guiding principles, and I am as empathetic and compassionate as I can be when listening to other's situations, mistakes, misfortunes... or what they perceive as errors in judgement. I encounter stories that are heart-wrenching to listen to, but I simply avoid

Walk In Faith & Medicine

judging them. It often feels like being in a confessional, where there is not much I can do but listen, and have a compassionate heart... These are moments in our practice that were not covered in Medical School - but were learned through 'on-the-job training'.

I often think it must be even more challenging for the patient when we know each other on a personal level. Especially given that they need my honest opinion and input in their gut-wrenching moment of time. Again, I do my best to be there for them, and guide best I can.

There are so many complicated matters surrounding the termination of pregnancy, and being on the frontline does not allow me to escape missiles being fired - whether they are from an opposing camp or even from a friendly one. I am fairly clear on the issues of rape and incest and the indication for termination. I don't think the principle of fairness can allow a pregnancy to continue in those situations... but ultimately, it is up to the mother to decide in all cases.

As practicing Obstetricians and Gynaecologists, we prescribe ultrasounds at regular intervals during the pregnancy. These are in large part to discern if there are any anatomical defects in the developing fetus with the main reason that we can inform the patient, and they can make a decision and have the option of continuing the pregnancy or not.

The one that gives me the most difficulty is the middle of the pregnancy - at twenty weeks. It's called an 'anatomical survey'. The results have to be explained to the patient. And in the case of gross anatomical

45

deformities (which are incompatible with life), the option of termination has to be known and offered to the patient. It is one of the primary reasons why the scan is strategically done at twenty weeks.

I remember a case during my residency where the sonogram at twenty weeks revealed an anencephalic fetus (baby developing without a head). The parents decided termination was not an option and carried the pregnancy to full term and delivered normally, with their expressed request, that everything should be done to save their baby. Despite all of this, the baby died shortly after separation from the mother. But their wishes were adhered to, and the parents seemed to have a sense of completion in following through with their decision.

The lines are blurred and probably more shades of grey than black or white, and I can't say that I know the right answer for the individuals.

After practicing in this field for over thirty-five years, I still have regular conflicts in decision-making. In trying to live a faith-based life, compassion is at the very heart of it all. The principle of doing unto others as you would have them do unto you, underlies my very being. I am certainly not infallible, and my conscience confronts me continually.

The issue of termination of pregnancy is an existential one for me, both personally and professionally, because of the work I do. I find solace in knowing that the Almighty is greater than our worried hearts and knows more about us than we do. I can't say I have found the answer, but I am guided in the hope that I'm at least on the right track in helping others along the way. I feel guided by the mystery of faith and trust, and it is in that conviction, I persevere.

Take one day at a time and the night will be rewarding –
Kedrick Pickering

JOURNAL 6

THE JOURNEY

Writing, for me, has long been an ambition that I have harbored. Dreaming about it and thinking about it, is in stark contrast to the idea of dreaming of becoming a physician in my teenage years. That dream would have been too gigantic for my limited brain at that time. Those were years when electricity was only minimally available in our community, and access to regional and international news was rare - if available at all. Recalling those days makes me think of an unseen presence that gave me hope.

The majority of the people I knew back then were anxiously awaiting relatives who lived overseas to file the documents for them to have their 'papers fixed'. This was the term used to describe the process of obtaining U.S. citizenship or a green card, which allowed people to migrate to the USA 'legally'. It was a badge of honor to obtain it, as the U.S. Virgin Islands next door beckoned with promises of the good life. The ones who were not so fortunate were like the forgotten ones left behind.

The nature of life in my community was not one of great economic prosperity, but there was a wealth of community. We learned to love, honor, respect and appreciate each other. We all understood that there was a presence greater than us, and again it gave us hope.

The chances of my family obtaining the coveted green card were minimal... So personally, there was not much hope placed on that possibility. It was more practical to focus on school in whatever capacity existed, as a more realistic pathway forward. These pathways were more likely to be in the area of education, primarily teaching or in government administration.

I well remember my father saying to me in a colloquial expression, "If you study your lesson, you'll become the government's own," meaning there was the possibility of 'going away' to school.

I was certainly encouraged in my primary school years by all my teachers. They all instilled in me the value of doing my best. I received several books as gifts, two of which I fondly recall: *The Student Companion* and *Animal Farm*. On my twelfth birthday, my mother gave me a Bible. It was a gift I wasn't particularly thrilled about at the time... "What is a 12-year-old kid to do with a Bible for a birthday gift?" I questioned myself! In retrospect however, it was probably fortuitous that a life of faith was being prophesied. I don't have any other gifts from when I was 12... but I still have that Bible.

The Bible and prayer were part of our daily diet. We prayed at home when we woke up, and again before we went to bed at night. We prayed in school in the morning before classes started. We had devotions. We prayed grace before meals, we prayed grace after meals, and we prayed before we departed from school in the afternoons.

In addition to the many times we attended church and prayed there, I would say we were well prayed up. How much that contributed to a life of faith is debatable, except that it exposed us to the greater good and to caring for our fellow man.

I can recall the many times in my medical life when my thoughts drifted back to those days. One patient I remember well was to undergo a major and potentially difficult surgery. During the pre-op preparation and visit with the patient, we went through the issues we were going to face. I guess it's fair to say there was apprehension in my words, and she sensed it.

The most reassuring words I could have heard at that moment might have been that my professor and mentor had just landed on the island and would join me in the operating room... But, no... that wasn't to be. Not even in my dreams. In fact, what I heard was even more profound and reassuring. She just quietly and confidently looked at me and said, "Doctor, let's do this. I will pray and you do the same."

It may sound unreal, but that surgery went as smoothly as could be, with no intraoperative or postoperative complications. Her recovery was completely uneventful.

My professor certainly wasn't there, but there was definitely a presence that brought a sense of serenity during that difficult time.

"Through the love of God the savior, all will be well."
Mary Peters

JOURNAL 7

COURAGE WITH PEACE

Mrs. Dally's unwavering faith in the face of her diagnosis taught me more about courage and resilience than any medical textbook ever could. She was an elderly woman when we met. I had been substituting for a colleague in his private practice while he was on vacation. She reminded me of my grandfather in many ways... They were both old-school, humble, God-fearing people with a dignity and confidence that belied their lowly status. They were from a generation where the economic conditions of the islands were poor at best.

Hers was a life of struggle for everyday survival, as was the case for most of the population. Growing up in the islands of the Caribbean in the early to mid-twentieth century, this was the lot of most. Daily bread was provided by daily work - relying primarily on the land and its produce to eke out a living. The weather and climatic conditions determined the quality of life. The kindness of nature was therefore solicited, primarily through faith and prayers to an Almighty and Loving

Father. In her and the older folks in the community, you saw a resilience and toughness that, no matter what, "My God will provide."

I recall that Mrs. Dally seemed delighted to meet a young doctor like myself. She seemed to have the belief that I would have the requisite knowledge to cure her aches and pains - most of which were associated with the aging process. Shortly into our conversation, however, it became apparent that this wasn't her primary concern. She was more focused on the simple hope that I, with my youth and enthusiasm, could offer some relief from the inevitable decline of old age.

A few consultations ensued, and we developed a bond. Her trust in me, the young doctor, and my respect for such a warm personality and a beautiful spirit, enhanced our friendship. She had weathered many storms in her life and always had a story to share with me about her trials and tribulations growing up on the islands.

However, the medical picture that began to emerge showed signs of a major storm brewing. The results of the various tests began to unfold, and the clinical picture was not very encouraging.

She was the matriarch of her close and extended family and a well-loved member of the community. She was well-respected and cared for by many, especially her niece, with whom she lived and would be accompanied to all her appointments. Mrs. Dally's health was not about to get better or even remain stable, for that matter. We had uncovered that she was suffering from a major illness, which was most likely terminal. It was gradually sapping her energy and strength away.

Everyone around her was concerned, and they were not prepared for their beloved Mrs. Dally to be in such a state. She had been a strong pillar of hope in her community for so long, that her sudden decline was difficult for many to accept.

The pressure mounted to refer her overseas for treatment, whatever and wherever it could be found. In our small community hospital, there was a recurrent need to transfer patients overseas for specialist medical care. However, Mrs. Dally had no insurance, and like most of the population, financial resources of that era were limited.

Above everything else, she had no desire to be transferred anywhere. She had spent her entire life in the small, quiet community of her birthplace, and she expressed to me quietly but confidently that if her time was up, she was prepared to die. She wanted to do so in familiar surroundings. She said to me, "Dr. Pickering the only place I want to be transferred to is into the arms of my Jesus."

With her wishes well-known to all concerned in her household, the family felt helpless as they witnessed her health continue to deteriorate. There was obvious weight loss and a loss of appetite. Mrs. Dally was becoming weaker and weaker.

The family and wider community found it increasingly burdensome and continued to insist on an overseas transfer. But Mrs. Dally stood firm and would have none of it. She was comfortable with the sense that her end was near and appeared quite at peace with it.

As her illness progressed, managing her care became increasingly challenging. The daily logistics of her care and travelling to and from the clinic were physically taxing. But even more challenging was answering the same questions repeatedly to various relatives. It became clear that another family meeting was necessary to explain the nature of her illness and the prognosis as a group. During the gathering, it was shared that the logistics of her care and the management of her pain were becoming overwhelming to the family. So, during that meeting, I volunteered to do home visits to ease their stress and help Mrs. Dally as much as possible.

Our bond had grown so deep in the short time I had known her, that I felt I had no choice but to give my all to alleviate her pain. It was painful for me, as a fellow human and member of the community, to see her in so much distress. Her pain had become her number one problem, but she steadfastly refused to be institutionalized. The nature of her pain required stronger and stronger medications - the kind that was worrisome to administer at home, especially during that time.

As her pain intensified, so did my own sense of helplessness. There came a point when I too needed comfort because this was new to me as a young physician. Normally in situations like this, patients are referred to specialists. But in the case of Mrs. Dally, my hands were tied. I wasn't prepared for how emotionally draining it was to watch her suffer and not step in with our usual protocol. But she remained firm in her decision and refused further care. I had to respect Mrs. Dally's autonomy and preserve her dignity. Through it all, she maintained a calm reassurance that everything would be well.

One day, about two days before she passed away, Mrs. Dally asked me to sit with her. The pain was clearly ravaging what remained of her frail body. She could barely muster the strength to speak. As I watched her struggle, my instinct was to reach for the narcotic analgesia I had on hand. But I had to honor her wishes, no matter how much it hurt me to do nothing. Finally, she found the strength to speak. As I leaned in close to her, she whispered, "Dr. Pickering, I don't want any more medicine. It's keeping me alive. I'm tired; I want to go home."

Her words stunned me. The silence between her bouts of pain was deafening, and the impact of her words was profound. At that moment, despite the agony she was enduring, she managed to smile - a radiant smile that melted my heart. It took everything in me not to break down in tears. I wasn't sure whether I was crying with her in celebration or in defeat.

She held my hand while squeezing it and whispered softly, "Thank you," as she drifted off to sleep. I placed her hand on her chest, tucked her in, and then left the room, feeling rather bewildered by what I had just witnessed.

That was the last time I saw Mrs. Dally alive. The next time I was called, I arrived too late - she had slipped away. Her family told me that in her final hours, her pain had become unbearable, but she refused even water. She was ready to leave this world and reassured them with her constant refrain: "It is well."

Healing I concluded, in some instances is finalized in physical death. Maybe, after all faith in an unseen being has a basis.

O let me hear thee speaking, In accents clear and still,
Above the storms of passion, the murmurs of self-will.
O speak to reassure me, to hasten or control,
O speak and make me listen, thou guardian of my soul -
John E Bode

JOURNAL 8

SCOULDING

I never expected that one conversation could change my life, but it did. Sister Bailey had witnessed the entire episode unfold from a spot where she remained completely unnoticed. I had no idea she'd seen anything until the moment she approached me and expressed her disappointment in my behavior. She referred me to the Book of Proverbs in the Bible quoting,

"Greater is he who rules his spirit than he who takes a city."

That quote marked the beginning of a meaningful conversation.

In the old English nursing tradition, the title "Sister" carries immense authority. Sister Bailey - though small in stature, was a towering figure in her profession. Her uniform was always spotless - lily-white with polished shoes, and she wore her red nurse's cap with distinction. This tradition, which sadly is no longer followed, was a clear symbol of leadership. There was no question about who was in charge.

In teaching institutions, the chain of command is crucial - much like in the military. It's a mark of respect among young professionals, including junior doctors, medical students, nursing students, and other health professionals on special rotations. Achieving the rank of a Sister, like Sister Bailey, was no small feat! She had certainly earned her place. People like her were the pillars of the healthcare profession, the keepers of records, and the standard-bearers. It wasn't uncommon to be rebuked by someone like Sister Bailey, often with the firm words, "Doctor, I can't believe what I just heard."

During my internship on the pediatric ward, I grew frustrated with one of the nurses. Whether I was right or wrong in my judgment is debatable, but my passion for the job got the best of me. I was harsh and disrespectful towards her - bordering on rude. Isaac Newton's law about every action having an equal and opposite reaction applied here, because the nurse's response was equally harsh and forceful. Our not-so-quiet disagreement quickly escalated into a heated argument - making everyone in the vicinity un-comfortable... including the parents visiting their sick children.

Suddenly, like a spirit, Sister Bailey appeared. The room fell silent. Both the nurse and I pretended to be busy, even exchanging awkward smiles. The nurse was quickly summoned to Sister Bailey's office with the dreaded words, "Nurse Smith can I see you in my office now?" When Sister Bailey said those words, you dropped everything and moved fast.

I was in even deeper trouble. What I had done was considered sacrilege in the medical field - being openly loud and disrespectful, especially in front of patients... not good. I knew I'd be reported to the professor and the head of the department. I expected no mercy and braced myself for the highest form of reprimand. I figured Sister Bailey would defend her nurse in front of the medical authorities. I had no defence.

However, Sister Bailey, with quiet dignity, acted as though she was merely passing by for her morning briefing. She discreetly pulled the nurse aside and invited her to the office. Then as if continuing on her way she approached me. In the softest voice, without even directly acknowledging me, she said, "Dr. Pickering I am very disappointed in you."

Ugh... my heart sank. If you've ever been scolded by someone you deeply respect, you understand the power of such words. I felt like the ground beneath me was giving way. My legs turned weak. I truly wished the earth would just swallow me whole.

Growing up, there was a saying: "Sticks and stones may break my bones, but words will never hurt me." That's one of the biggest lies. Sister Bailey's words might as well have pierced my heart with a dagger! The weight of rejection and shame was crushing, all due to my prideful behavior.

Sister Bailey wasn't in my presence for more than 90 seconds, but it felt like an eternity. I was trembling, fearing what would happen next. I expected her to report me to the higher-ups, and I dreaded the consequences. But instead, with her calm and motherly demeanor, she repeated the words,

"Greater is he who rules his spirit than he who takes a city,"

and then the Sister urged me to find the passage in the Bible. Without further fuss, she quietly went on her way.

What I didn't know at the time was that Sister Bailey attended the same church I did. Later on, during another interaction, she mentioned how impressed she was to see a young, busy doctor like me making time for church. It didn't matter to her what my motivations were - she was pleased to see me there. This only reinforced her disappointment in my behavior that day.

To my great relief, Sister Bailey didn't report the incident to anyone. She was as proper in her demeanor as she was in her appearance… embodying the values of the Florence Nightingale era of nursing. She held herself and her profession in the highest regard and wanted to pass down those traditions to the next generation.

God-fearing in her ways, Sister Bailey's rebuke was delivered with wisdom and grace, imparted through the sayings of Solomon. If I had been disciplined by the medical authorities, the punishment wouldn't have been as life-altering as the softly spoken words of Sister Bailey.

Since that day, whenever I'm faced with potentially explosive situations, I pause and reflect before acting impulsively. All thanks to the Sister's gentle but powerful correction. The quiet words she spoke that morning left an indelible mark on my consciousness.

This small, unassuming woman, with her calm temperament and commanding presence, taught me one of life's most important lessons... and for that, I am forever grateful.

"Faith is the bird that feels the light and sings when the dawn is still dark.'
Ravindranath Tagore

JOURNAL 9

YES OR NO?

Every morning as I don my white coat, I'm reminded that my true purpose lies not just in healing bodies but in nurturing souls. It's interesting how this mantra has become even more deliberate with the passage of time.

In the past, imparting knowledge to younger patients came naturally. Now, as I grow older, I do so with more conscious intent.

The challenge lies in balancing this approach; there's always the risk of being overly intrusive. When dealing with obvious disorders like hypertension or diabetes, the conversation is straightforward. But with more personal issues, the challenge can create disharmony if not handled delicately.

Confrontation is something to avoid, especially on sensitive matters. We live in a world where we make all kinds of investments, sometimes forgetting our health or being unaware of the consequences of an unhealthy lifestyle. There's a responsibility to encourage healthy living and foster a better understanding of health.

The World Health Organization (WHO) defines health as "not just the absence of disease, but the complete mental, social, psychological, physical, emotional and spiritual well-being of the individual." This is a tall order for healthcare professionals who truly want to promote healthy living, but it's a worthy effort.

I recall my experience with Mrs. W. She had been separated from her husband and involved in another relationship. Her estranged husband was similarly involved with someone else, but they weren't legally divorced.

She became pregnant and had a normal pregnancy, labor and delivery. Life continued. She attended all her regular post-delivery check-ups, and we had family planning discussions.

A few months later, she visited my office for non-medical reasons. She needed some passport documents and pictures of the baby signed. This was a common request and there was nothing unusual about the visit; I had likely done it for her two other children. However, this time the details were different. She wanted the child's documents to reflect her husband's name, for reasons personal to her. This surprising request put me in a very uncomfortable position.

There was a long, pregnant pause in our interaction. She asked if something was wrong, sensing my hesitation. After what felt like an eternity, I responded nervously, asking if she realized what she was asking me to do. Her response, tinged with surprise, was a genuine "no".

I then asked if she understood that what she was requesting was dishonest and unethical. Again, surprised she asked, "In what way doctor?"

The conversation took a tense turn. I pointed out nervously and sheepishly so as not to offend her, that we both knew her husband was not the father. For me to sign a document using his name would be dishonest, legally and morally wrong.

You could have knocked her over with a feather. The look of total embarrassment and immediate remorse was palpable. She started to cry… sobbing uncontrollably. It took everything in me to console her and bring her back to a position of control. In those moments, I felt as if I had done something immensely wrong, dishonoring or disrespecting her. We were both in a very awkward and uncomfortable place, at least for a few moments.

When she regained her composure, she apologized profusely. Her response shocked me. As if I had been awakened suddenly from a deep sleep. It took a few seconds to comprehend her words, which still resonate with me today.

She taught me one of the most profound lessons of my life. Her words - "Dr. Pickering," she paused, almost exasperated, and then continued, "people don't run from a good thing." I was blown away, pausing to let those words penetrate my inner being.

She continued, "If my husband had treated me well, I would have had no reason to leave. I had to run for my life."

For the next several minutes, she shared excruciating details of her life - of the mental, physical and emotional abuse she had endured. She spoke as if to an audience, revealing the deep wounds caused by this abuse. Her words were intermingled with moments of sobbing and despair. I sat and listened - as a therapist would. With each new detail she revealed, I could feel the pain she had experienced. As if watching it unfold in real-time.

She apologized repeatedly for putting me in such an embarrassing position and thanked me for listening and pointing out the extent of her request, which to her was innocent. I felt the sincerity in her apology and acknowledged my own misgivings and any additional hurt I might have caused in my initial response.

In my reflections, I was pleased that I had been respectful in my response. I did not belittle or dehumanize her, and I was proud of this after the outcome of such an open dialogue.

I found her words impactful!

"People don't run from a good thing"...

Wow! The depth of empathy that we both encountered, still remains inexplicable to me today.

As lessons in life go, this one ranks in the top tier of my journey. We never know what others are going through; everyone has a story, if only we're willing to listen. No one runs from a good thing.

In my journey of faith, I compare this to encountering the Man from Galilee… It's difficult to run away from a relationship with Him once you've been introduced to Him.

"The power of faith can create miracles in healing."
Anonymous

JOURNAL 10

MIRACULOUS RECOVERY

The signs were ominous. She had been diagnosed with a tumor on her ovary. She was 32 years old and presented with severe lower abdominal pain, looking and feeling profoundly unwell. She appeared pale - white as a sheet - with a cachectic appearance. All indications pointed to advanced ovarian cancer.

The clinical picture demanded urgent intervention. At a minimum, we had to alleviate her pain. The year was 1994. There were only two of us surgeons and we lacked advanced investigative tools. There was no MRI or CT scan, and our laboratory facilities were minimal at best. Her pain was intense, and surgery seemed inevitable. The ultrasound confirmed a large pelvic mass but provided limited details.

Complicating matters further she had no medical insurance, was not a local resident and her passport had expired. Referral to an overseas centre for optimal care wasn't an option. She required a multi-disciplinary team approach to assess for metastatic disease, which could have shifted management to palliative care.

Initial lab results revealed severe anemia, with a blood count about one-quarter of the normal level (4.6 mg/dL). This explained her pallor and overall weakness. However, our hospital had no active blood bank. Instead, we operated a "walk-in bank," calling donors as needed. I recall one gentleman who had donated blood around seventy times due to the high demand for his rare blood type. His generosity likely saved many lives.

Unfortunately, this patient had no extended family to assist with donating blood, creating both logistical and medical challenges. Without a transfusion, surgery was out of the question. A major medical disaster loomed.

This was not a case I could manage alone, especially given our limited resources. Postoperative care ideally required a fully equipped intensive care unit. Puerto Rico, our referral center, just sixty miles away, might as well have been a world away. I fervently wished someone else could handle this case, but I had no choice. I had to dig deep and rely on what little faith I had.

My initial conversation with her revealed a scared, anxious young woman. Her expression mirrored my own apprehension. Despite my professional facade, my concern about her prognosis was difficult to conceal.

We needed to operate, but not without first securing a blood transfusion. I explained the urgency to her and then rushed to the lab to emphasize the situation. The walk-in blood bank was activated with frantic calls to regular donors, who, in turn, spread the word. The local Red Cross also mobilized its network.

I consulted with my surgical colleague, a seasoned friend and mentor. Together, we reviewed the patient's case and shared the same grave concerns about the risks of intervention. It was one of those dilemmas where not operating meant certain death, but surgery might hasten her demise.

Her limited support system stepped up, including a cousin and her church family. While their presence initially felt intrusive, their efforts in finding blood donors proved invaluable. With transfusions underway, we could finally set a timeline for surgery. Her pain was worsening and the anesthesiologist warned that further delays increased the risk of a poor outcome.

Before surgery, I addressed the 'family' to explain the plan and risks. It was nerve-wracking to tell them that this might be their last time seeing her alive. The prognosis was at best fifty-fifty. The tension was palpable.

About seven of us stood by her bedside - medical staff and family members - when someone asked if we could pray together. While I had often heard promises of prayer, this was the first time I was asked to join in. Feeling awkward, I agreed.

I don't remember the exact words, but phrases like "bless the hands of the nurses and doctors" and "Thy will be done" stood out.

What followed was an indescribable sense of peace and reassurance. A calm settled over us, and we proceeded with renewed focus.

The surgery was a daunting six-hour ordeal. The pelvic mass was bleeding, and all surrounding structures were matted together - making the anatomy nearly indiscernible. Several times the temptation to "open and close" loomed, but we pressed on... guided by an inexplicable sense of assurance.

She received two units of blood during surgery, in addition to the four units preoperatively. Despite numerous challenges, there were no complications. Each obstacle felt surmountable, as though an unseen hand guided us.

When she awoke and was transferred to recovery, relief swept through the team. Her recovery was uneventful, and she was discharged on the seventh postoperative day. Bright, cheerful and with color in her cheeks, she was the embodiment of gratitude.

I saw her twice for follow-ups... each time marvelling at her transformation. At six weeks, she was almost unrecognizable - radiant, well-dressed and smiling. She thanked everyone at the clinic, even leaving flowers and thank-you cards for the nurses and surgeons.

I never saw her again, as she likely migrated shortly after.

This case has stayed with me... a testament to the words of St. Augustine:

"Pray as though everything depended on God.

Work as though everything depended on you."

When faith is present, work must follow."

The mind has great influence over the body, and
maladies often have their origin there."
Maimonides

JOURNAL 11

UNINTENDED
CONSEQUENCES

Looking back now, I realize that every decision I made
was a step toward finding my true self. Like most
youngsters of the sixties, seventies and eighties, I had
my share of personal and cultural struggles. We were
the children of the era of the civil rights movement in
the U.S.A… the independence movement in the
Caribbean, and further afield, the apartheid era in
Southern Africa. Being a medical student did not make
me immune to the sociocultural issues of the day.

We grew up on a diet of revolutionary expression - in
thoughts, words and sometimes action. It was a clash
between traditional medical education and expressions
of anti-establishment verbiage, as in the words of
Robert (Bob) Nesta Marley, one of the most popular
artists of the day…

"Rise up and live."

Learning to live in this environment created its own dynamics, and it can well be imagined that there were inherent conflicts. The conservative mode of dress was challenged at one's own risk - almost suicidal to your medical career. Freedom of thought was acceptable; freedom of expression was an entirely different story. My hairstyle and beard were tolerated, but were considered somewhat unconventional.

I recall one of my professors, in a curious sort of way, asking if my appearance was part of my religion. I was somewhat taken aback, as it indeed was not. But I soon came to understand that he was genuinely interested in finding out. I didn't think he was being intimidating in his curiosity, nor did I feel he was suggesting anything inappropriate. It was however, an eye-opener - a revealing conversation.

Participation in that dialogue showed me that sometimes in life, confirmation is vital and essential to achieving bigger goals. Outward appearance doesn't always convey who your inner self truly is. I recognized that my professor was giving me a life lesson not found in textbooks. He candidly and courteously shared the following insight:

"No one will complain to you about your dress code; they just won't allow you to pass your course."

His words hit me hard. I had long struggled with my faith and its expression, and this was one of those priceless lessons not found in textbooks. I continued to seek guidance from the unseen hand and resolved not to let my revolutionary thoughts sabotage my medical school journey.

Of course, I modified my grooming and went on to complete my medical degree. My enthusiasm and commitment to becoming the best physician I could be were tested on several occasions… but each experience taught me valuable lessons.

One such occasion occurred during my internship. It was my weekend off, but the ward rounds had to be completed on Saturday morning, and patients were handed over to the doctor on duty. I was hurrying to finish my rounds; the sooner this was done, the earlier I could leave for some much-needed relaxation.

I remember feeling excited about the day and evening ahead - there was something special awaiting me after work. I was bubbling with joy and anticipation, but I must have inadvertently done or said something to offend one of the nurses. I cannot recall any specific action or remark that would warrant a formal complaint to the nursing supervisor, but that's what ensued. Without informing me that I had caused any offence, the nurse brought the supervisor to chastise me.

Without any inquiry or making me aware of what transgression I had committed, the nursing supervisor confronted me with harsh words. She proceeded to tell me, "I am going to fix your business." These were fighting words to which I dared not respond, particularly since I was clueless as to what I had done wrong. I was genuinely confused.

I felt as if I had been accused, tried, and sentenced in a court, where I hadn't even been read the charges. I had committed the most heinous of medical crimes yet remained painfully unaware of what it was. Lost and bewildered, I began questioning myself about what would happen next. Self-pity became my companion - I had no other - and I didn't know where to turn. A promising weekend suddenly appeared bleak, as if a storm warning had just been issued. I imagined facing the Supreme Court of the hospital without a defense.

I prayed to God Almighty, hoping He would send an angel to stand in the gap for me. I knew I wasn't a favorite of the supervisor, but even that offered no solace. I couldn't fathom what I could have done that was so abominable.

As expected, the Consultant Obstetrician on duty showed up for rounds. I was quaking in my boots. No sooner had he appeared on the ward than the nursing supervisor pulled him aside to complain about me. It was done in such a way that it was obvious she was reporting something serious. The Consultant's gaze focused on me with an intensity that could have melted snow on a mountain.

By then, I felt as if my hospital contract and medical career were over. These were after all the crème de la crème of the hospital establishment. My goose was cooked, and I wasn't even invited to the party. I wanted to pray for divine intervention, but words failed me.

In what I would describe as the final act, the Consultant approached me sternly and asked, "Dr. Pickering, what time do you think you'll be finished with the rounds?" I replied in a quaking voice, "In about an hour, Sir." He nodded, paused, and then commanded, "Well, I want to see you in my office right after." As he departed, he added, "I'll be waiting for you." The nursing supervisor smiled at me in a way that suggested, "Take that."

I hurriedly completed my tasks, avoiding her and the other nurse as if they were the plague. Taking care of patients in such a tense environment was nearly impossible; my enthusiasm for the day had evaporated.

Heading to the Consultant's office, I felt my anxiety grow. My heartbeat thundered in my chest and for a moment, I thought I was having a heart attack. I dreaded being found guilty of something unknown to me and expected the harshest of sentences - suspension followed by termination.

The unseen hand must have heard my cry. To my surprise, the Consultant greeted me warmly... offering tea and biscuits. He invited me to sit on the couch and engaged me in a genuine conversation about my internship and future plans. After fifteen minutes he rose and said with a smile, "Dr. Pickering... in life sometimes justice has to appear to have been done, even if it is not." He shook my hand, wished me a happy weekend, and encouraged me to keep up the good work.

He never mentioned the supervisor's complaint and I didn't ask. I have since concluded that guardian angels do exist, protecting us from harm. As I left his office, I exhaled deeply, and the day seemed brighter again.

Faith is being sure of that which we hope for.
It is being sure of what we do not see."
Hebrews 11:1

JOURNAL 12

TERMINAL ILLNESS

Observing Mr. Green's demeanor and his steadfast belief in a higher power (even as he faced a terminal illness) profoundly reshaped my attitude toward patient care. Fresh from medical school and armed with a wealth of facts and figures and an understanding of current research trends - I felt invincible. I recall one of our professors telling us, as we prepared for our final exams, that we were at a point where we would know as much about general medicine as we ever would. Knowing the latest treatment options and their applications is crucial to medical practice, and it was always impressive to hear our professors command the profession with such authority in the university setting.

During a teaching round with the professor, residents, interns, medical students and nurses - the hierarchy was clear: each of us sought to impress with our knowledge. Mr. Green, the patient at whose bedside we stood, had recently been diagnosed with cancer but had not yet been informed. The prognosis was poor, and it was up to the junior staff to discuss the test results with him.

This had to be done truthfully while still offering hope for successful treatment. After all, the university setting is designed to provide the latest and most effective treatment modalities.

Mr. Green had limited family support, with most of his visitors being his pastor and fellow church members. It was crucial to share his test results with him directly and humanely, especially in the absence of family. We understood our responsibility to provide hope for healing and recovery, but despite our best efforts, what happened next was nothing short of extraordinary.

As we made rounds, eight of us gathered at his bedside to discuss his management. Mr. Green appeared unaware of our presence, seemingly asleep. When he eventually awoke and became aware of us, he asked, "Doctor what did you say...that I have cancer?" The entire room and his demeanor shifted dramatically.

None of us had directly told him he had cancer, so his reaction was unexpected. The word 'cancer' had been mentioned indirectly in our discussion about obtaining help from the cancer society and involving a social worker. We had been discussing his social circumstances in a general manner, never imagining he was paying close attention or understanding all that was said.

The following day, as I attended to my usual tasks on the ward and visited his bedside, I sensed a change in him. He seemed distant, and our interaction felt uncomfortable. I found myself facing him after not directly using the term 'cancer', feeling as though I had been deceitful.

We are trained to be as tactful as possible when revealing a difficult diagnosis and to allow the process to unfold gradually. In some cases, family members are given the diagnosis and then communicate it to the patient, based on the specific situation to avoid undue distress.

My interaction with Mr. Green during this visit was revealing. The room took on a different atmosphere. His face shone brightly with a serene smile, almost angelic, as if he were in a peaceful place.

He spoke softly, and the two of us present listened intently. "Doctor," he said, "I was in a faraway place and I saw little children, all smiling, happy and singing. They were dressed in white and beckoning me with outstretched hands to come." His countenance was peaceful, and he appeared to be in a state of profound tranquility.

He smiled again, closed his eyes and drifted off to sleep, leaving us to wonder what we had just witnessed. I pondered these things in my heart, trying to understand the profound peace he seemed to experience despite facing a terminal illness.

Mr. Green's treatment, as decided by the medical team, continued daily as he prepared to start a course of cancer treatment. Despite his apparent detachment and lack of interest in the planned treatment, he remained pleasant and content, never complaining.

He quietly passed away during a daytime nap, his face adorned with a serene smile. The nurse discovered his passing only during her routine checks.

Although Mr. Green seldom spoke about his beliefs, he lived them through his daily interactions. He came alive when his church brethren visited, and he appeared joyful during those times. I don't recall him ever asking about his discharge from the hospital. In retrospect, he likely knew about his eternal home and that his time was near.

"Where love lives, fear cannot exist."
Carrie Kohan

JOURNAL 13

FAITH IN ACTION

"Are you sure you can do this? Are you going to be alright?" my wife Alice asked as she was being wheeled into the operating room.

"You can't have faith and not have faith," I replied. This was a saying we often shared with one another during difficult situations - this was no different! And when I think back to this time and how brave she was, it still amazes me that my wife cared more about how I was feeling, than about herself.

Alice's pregnancy had been uneventful. The test results and the only ultrasound performed were all normal. We are people of faith and trusted that everything would go well. My dear beloved, in particular, has an abiding faith that is often difficult for me to comprehend - during the pregnancy, this was even more evident. Alice believed and trusted she was safe, and that belief alone was enough to keep me encouraged.

My surgical colleague kept me up to date throughout the entire pregnancy and during labor. We were mindful of the ethics involved in my role as both husband and doctor. Normally, this dual role is not allowed, but the harsh reality was that I was the only practicing obstetrician at the hospital on our island at the time. To ensure we followed protocol, I consulted with my former professor at the University Hospital, where I had worked regularly. Monitoring the pregnancy was straightforward, as there were no complications - at least not yet.

Labor began normally, around the expected due date. My wife was monitored by the midwives with their usual care and diligence. Alice herself was a nurse and midwife, so her colleagues, with whom she worked daily, surrounded her in anticipation. There was an air of excitement and extra energy in the ward. Two of her closest colleagues and friends stayed throughout the labor and decided to be present for the delivery.

Normally, a husband would sit with his wife, awaiting the arrival of their blessed child together. However, because I might become her emergency physician, I had to pace the corridors - trying to keep myself occupied while waiting with bated breath for news of the delivery of our baby, and my family's health.

Anxiety was high because this was our first child. It was also the first time I was on the opposite side of the delivery table. This pivotal day gave my practice a whole new sense of meaning. For the first time, I could relate to every father or loved one pacing the corridors… feeling helpless to alleviate their partner's pain and discomfort.

I reflected on many past patients and the strength of each woman as she gave birth. I recalled the overwhelming awe in their spouses' eyes as they witnessed the miracle of life. Some tears were of joy and celebration, while others were of loss and anguish.

Having seen the risks firsthand, I prayed relentlessly for the health of my wife and our little one. For hours, I paced, unable to sit still. I wanted to be there. I wanted to help, but protocol demanded I wait. And wait, I did.

Eventually, I found a small, wooden couch in a stark hallway. Exhausted, I sat down, bent over and put my face in my hands, and prayed: "Please dear Lord, hold my family in Your loving hands and bring them through this birth with Your grace."

Memories of the past and worry must have been evident on my face because the head nurse came over to check on me. I was touched by the love and concern the team had for both Alice and me. Feeling complete in my prayer, I attempted to rest. Lying awkwardly on the small couch, my long legs hung over one side, while my head rested against the hard wooden arm.

Doctors learn during training to fall asleep in awkward places, even if it's just for a few minutes. I must have drifted off because I woke with a jolt in the early hours of the morning. I panicked, thinking I had missed my child's birth!

I got up and ran to the nurses' desk, where I learned

Alice's labor was still progressing ever so slowly. After twenty-four hours with no progress over the last eight, contractions were waning. Under normal circumstances, this would have been a straightforward decision to deliver by Caesarean section, but this wasn't a normal situation. The senior midwife, someone I deeply respected, pulled me aside and said it was time to intervene. She spoke with quiet authority, giving me the reassurance I needed to make the decision.

I consulted my professor and surgical colleague. Both agreed with the decision and offered their support. As I scrubbed for surgery, I pushed aside fear. Creator was with me.

When Alice was wheeled into the operating room, her hand reached out to me and our eyes met for the first time in hours. I kissed her and reassured her. Her concern was less for herself and more for me - even in her condition! This touched my heart deeply.

The surgery was uneventful, but I'll never forget the moment the midwife exclaimed, "It's a boy!" Joy and relief swept over all of us in the OR. And as I sewed the last suture, the realization sank in… My family was safe. We had a son.

Looking into Alice's eyes, I whispered, "We have a boy... You did it my love." Tears of joy filled both our eyes as we celebrated this incredible moment together.

As the years have passed, I'm often asked what it was like delivering my own children. I usually reply, "Life gives us challenges, and we have to step up." Yet, deep down, I know the truth: it was faith that carried us through.

Reflecting on that day, I've come to understand the profound meaning of...

"Faith without works is dead."

It wasn't just my hands that delivered our son - it was faith in action, and an unseen hand guiding us throughout the way.

This day remains one of the greatest blessings of my life, a true testament to walking in faith.

Show me your faith apart from your works, and
I by my works will show you, my faith."
James 2:18

JOURNAL 14

DILIGENT PRAYER

As I scrubbed in for surgery, I whispered a prayer - not
just for steady hands but for wisdom, courage and the
best possible outcome. "Would we, could we, save this
life?"

It had been a particularly long and tiresome day on all
fronts: work, home, and the usual everyday chores.
After completing my evening rounds and ensuring that
all the patients on the ward were stable, I was looking
forward to getting home and settling in for a restful
night. Home beckoned, and I longed for the comfort of
laying down the burdens of the day.

This was a time before mobile phones and pagers. It
was during a period of time when I was the only
practicing obstetrician/gynaecologist at the community
hospital.

For about eight years, my sole surgical backup was my general surgeon colleague. We were the only two people in the hospital who could perform surgeries, and in real emergencies, our expertise often had to extend beyond our comfort zones. If time didn't allow for a transfer outside the country, we had no choice. We were each other's support and companions in every sense.

When I arrived home, I was greeted with a note to call the hospital immediately. My dear wife, a nurse herself, handed the piece of paper to me with a look of concern. The tone of her voice made it clear that time wasn't on my side. "Wow!" I thought. "This can't be real." Dutifully, I dialed the hospital. The words on the other end were chilling: "Come quickly. Mrs. Jones is bleeding and it's heavy!"

My heart skipped a beat. This was the same patient I had seen about twenty minutes earlier and had discharged to go home. The only reason she hadn't physically left was because she lived on another island, and there was no transportation available until the following day. The phone nearly slipped from my hand as a wave of panic and dread washed over me. I instructed the nurse on immediate measures to take while I gathered the mental and physical strength to head back to the hospital.

Mixed emotions were my constant companion as I drove. I was scared, anxious and distressed. In my mind, I cursed every driver who was in my way - wishing they would all disappear. I prayed for the nurse's competence and guidance, and I prayed for safe passage. Despite my best efforts, the journey felt endless.

When I finally arrived, Mrs. Jones was still actively bleeding, despite the nurse's near-perfect execution of my instructions. She was on her third post-operative day, recovering well after an uneventful cesarean section. Her discharge had been in order, and I often wonder what her fate would have been if she had left the hospital that evening. Would she have made it back in time? Situations like this force reflection on the unseen hand working in our favor.

Our immediate efforts to stop the hemorrhage were only partially successful. Reoperation was the last thing I wanted after such a long day, but as the bleeding persisted, we had no choice. We had to find the source, likely a burst suture, and move quickly.

With fear gnawing at me and my strength waning, I called my surgical colleague for assistance. Even with help on the way, I felt utterly drained, both physically and emotionally. As I scrubbed in for surgery, I realized how depleted of food and rest I was. Prayer was my only remaining option. I asked for divine help, not just assistance, and I believe my prayer was heard.

Emergencies like this never feel fast enough. Every moment feels like an eternity. Anxiety gripped the room as we searched for the source of the bleeding. Then, I heard the head nurse, a woman of immense faith, praying quietly in the background as she diligently assisted. Her quiet prayers brought a sense of reassurance to the team.

We soon reached a critical juncture: remove Mrs. Jones's womb or risk losing her on the table. It was a life-altering decision, but there was no alternative. Once the decision was made, the procedure proceeded smoothly. By the end, the operating room was quiet, a palpable sense of peace settling over everyone. We breathed a collective sigh of relief and gratitude. Even those who didn't consider themselves people of faith remarked, "God was on our side."

Perhaps the most astonishing part of this case was Mrs. Jones's reaction post-operatively. She told me she had been praying diligently for me and the team, right up until she was put under anesthesia. She said she had noticed our worry but had an unshakable peace that everything would be alright.

Mrs. Jones recovered well. She continued to express gratitude to the staff and became an ongoing source of inspiration for us all. Her words, "joyful and grateful" became a mantra that resonated deeply. It's difficult not to be moved by someone like her, someone who truly embodies Ralph Waldo Emerson's words:

"I'd rather see a sermon than hear one."

O safe to the rock that is higher than I
My soul in its conflicts and sorrows would fly."
William O Cushing

JOURNAL 15

PAIN AND JOY

Traversing the nature and complexities of my patient's medical ailments brought me to a place of personal conflict. We, as medical students, were young and impressionable, full of enthusiasm and ready to change the world. But so were many of our patients! They were the same age as many of us who were caring for them.

There was an unspoken belief that we were not supposed to get sick or afflicted with such chronic and debilitating illnesses at our young age. These were degenerative disorders after all, that were reserved for those more advanced in years… or so we thought. It all seemed so unfair, especially when listening to the professor give such a grave and poor prognosis to someone who could have been a friend in school. This was, after all, the University Hospital, with the brightest and best doctors who knew it all; we expected only positive outcomes as freshly released medical students. Little did we know that our education was just beginning...

As interns, we were assigned to individual patients - two of us to each patient. This was a part of the orientation and learning process. We were expected to know every-thing about the person, the medical illness and all the possible modalities of treatment. It meant spending extended periods of time with the patient, and in the process, we were to establish a professional bond with respectable bedside manners. Being young and anxious to learn, I wanted to impress the professor with clinical knowledge, but it was also difficult to not become close to the patient and their families, nor be swept away in their situations. Over time, of course, you learn to separate the range of human emotions, but that was not the case early on, in our careers.

Our young patient was suffering from a rare, debilitating autoimmune disorder, the science of which was far from understood in the nineteen-eighties. There were a range of clinical beliefs that were changing on a regular basis. Every time there seemed to be light at the end of the tunnel, that tunnel suddenly became dark again - like a mirage.

Being closely associated with the patient, we were confronted with the hard questions. There were no direct and encouraging answers, and we often felt helpless and dejected. This wasn't how it was supposed to be... we were the ones meant to give answers and cures, or so we thought.

And with the passing of time, even more perplexing

situations were created. The ailment itself was new to science; the knowledge base was unfolding, as there was precious little research already done in the area. In fact, one of our senior colleagues with whom we worked at that time eventually went on to international fame from the research he did in this area. Looking back, it is so discomforting that our abilities in this regard were extremely limited.

But immunology is now a well-researched and better-understood area of medicine. Thankfully, autoimmune disorders are better and more often successfully treated now. That wasn't the case with our young patient back in the early 1980s. Her illness was rapidly progressive - depleting her of the ability to fight. She developed what is now, in retrospect, almost all of the major complications of this disorder.

We watched helplessly from the sidelines as she deteriorated and eventually passed away. Medicine was not at the position it is today. There was nothing we could offer, but comfort…

About six weeks after a fellow intern and I had come to know her, she slipped away. She was fifteen years old and passed away on a day when both of us were not around to assist in her departure. I vividly recall the emotional turmoil when we arrived on the ward the following day. We both headed to her bedside, only to discover that it was empty. The emptiness was palpable… even now.

As I relive those terrible moments. We hadn't yet been taught about death and dying in any meaningful way;

we hadn't been exposed to the deeper intellectual methods of grief and the grief reaction. This wasn't how it was supposed to have ended. It was devastating not only for her family, but for the both of us as well.

I was left bewildered and heartbroken. "Where was God in all of this? Did He not care? How could He let our patient die? Why didn't we find the cure or at least some intervention to slow the progress of the disease?"

A young life, not yet blossomed, gone far too soon - it seemed so unfair. My search for answers here was one of the first major conflicts I had with faith and medicine. This was a personal struggle; there weren't any such open discussions taking place. Medicine wasn't a profession for weak souls.

We attended the funeral in our small community and grieved as best we could with her family. My journey of faith in my professional life was in its embryonic stage. There was still a long way to go.

"Even children are known by the way they act, whether their conduct is pure and whether it is right."
Proverbs 20:11

JOURNAL 16

RESPECT FOR AUTONOMY

Many see faith and science as opposites. But in my journey, they have become harmonious companions. The patient who had just been seated, accompanied by her husband, appeared troubled. Right away, she told me she was feeling unwell. She also mentioned she had been referred by one of her elders and that she was a Jehovah's Witness. That was critical information. Her main issue was persistent bleeding for about six weeks, coupled with a general malaise or discomfort.

It was late on a Friday afternoon, the end of the workweek. The nurse at my surgery informed me about a new patient, who had no appointment and looked ill. Selfishly, I have to admit, it wasn't what I wanted to hear at that hour... but I had to compose myself and put on my best professional demeanor. I knew the week wasn't going to end as planned.

The couple, both in their early thirties, had been

married less than two years and had no children. The bleeding pattern was a significant concern as they were contemplating starting a family. They had sought help elsewhere - trying various treatments with limited success. By the time they arrived at our surgery, they were desperate for answers.

I was in a quandary. The treatment protocols she had already received were appropriate, but none had yielded positive results. The next logical step - one that seemed almost inevitable - would likely require a blood transfusion. However, this was in contraindication to her faith.

The lab was about to close, but I managed to obtain a blood count. The results confirmed the clinical picture: she was severely anemic, with a hemoglobin level of 5.8 g/dL. There was no choice but to refer her for hospitalization under our care.

Two competing narratives presented themselves: it was the weekend, resources were limited, and the patient would not accept blood transfusions. This was a peculiar predicament. In small institutions like ours, managing medical issues often comes hand-in-hand with navigating interpersonal and professional conflicts, which can take on a life of their own.

Voltaire once said,

"Faith consists in believing when it is beyond the power of reason to believe."

Reflecting on this, I realized that philosophical resolve

and my own faith were not just important but essential. This was a patient on the brink of collapse, requiring the best of us - not the worst. Time was not on our side, and there was no room for confusion or hesitation.

A subtle resistance arose among some healthcare team members, fueled by discomfort with differing religious beliefs. Managing this dynamic was crucial to prevent unnecessary friction. Questions surfaced: How do we manage a patient actively bleeding, unwilling to accept blood transfusions, and for whom surgery was not an immediate option? And what if the bleeding worsened?

I recalled an experience during my residency. A male patient, injured in a motor vehicle accident, needed emergency surgery and a blood transfusion. Outside the operating room, a conflict erupted between family members - some were Jehovah's Witnesses, others not. The decision was urgent, tensions ran high, and security had to intervene. Ultimately, the spouse relented and authorized the transfusion. The patient survived and was discharged with a positive prognosis. That memory underscored the ethical complexities we now faced.

Our current patient was anxious and scared. We had extensive discussions about her condition, potential management options, and the direction we recommended. The immediate priority was stopping the bleeding. Yet most treatments had already been tried unsuccessfully, raising the possibility of a rare underlying disorder.

Her elder visited at her request, reinforcing her stance

against blood transfusions. Intravenous fluids and iron supplementation were permissible, along with alternative therapies. Once we all agreed on an acceptable protocol, I prescribed a medical regimen that I had used during my residency. The staff was understandably apprehensive.

To everyone's relief, the bleeding slowed after 48 hours and stopped completely by the fourth day. Without further bleeding, it would take three to four months for her blood count to normalize with continued iron and vitamin supplementation. During this time, she faced significant physical limitations.

Investigations revealed that she had uterine fibroids - a common condition in women of African descent. Treatment for fibroids typically involves surgery, but we had to wait for her anemia to resolve. Fortunately, newer medications could suppress her menstrual cycle, halting the bleeding and allowing her blood count to recover. Only then could we plan for a major operation - a myomectomy - to remove the fibroids, a procedure notorious for blood loss.

This created another dilemma. Anesthesiologists typically require that blood be available for transfusion during such surgeries. However, given her beliefs, this wasn't an option. We outlined the risks, and she accepted them, prepared to move forward when the time came.

Four months later, her blood count had returned to normal. Before proceeding with surgery, we had further discussions with the couple and her elders, who consulted their headquarters in the United States. They arranged for a shipment of alternative intravenous products acceptable to their faith.

By the time surgery day arrived, spirits were high, and the team was confident. All necessary protocols to minimize blood loss were in place. The patient was otherwise healthy, with no anaesthetic risks beyond the potential for blood loss.

Plato's words came to mind:

"We are twice armed if we fight with faith."

The surgery lasted four hours, with average blood loss and no major complications. Her recovery in the postoperative unit was smooth, and the nursing staff breathed a collective sigh of relief. The mood across the team was jubilant.

During her recovery, a steady stream of visitors - family, friends, and fellow congregants, filled her room. Observing from a distance, I marveled at how faith can influence outcomes. I pondered the words,

"For those who believe, all things are possible."

Thomas Aquinas also said,

"To one who has faith, no explanation is necessary.

To one without faith, no explanation is possible."

This experience reaffirmed the many facets of responsibility we bear as caregivers... responsibilities steeped in faith, respect, and unwavering commitment to our patients.

"Your words and thoughts are your fingerprints on the universe."
Carrie Kohan

JOURNAL 17

INNOCENCE

What do you do when, with the best intentions in the world, your decision lands you embroiled in a major debacle?

My patient, who was 38 years old, had an uneventful pregnancy, labor, and delivery of her third child. She and her spouse had already decided that this would be their last and were prepared to have a 'tie-off' (Bilateral Tubal Ligation). We thought we'd cleared all the necessary hurdles, and we had agreed to do the procedure post-delivery or, if we had to perform an emergency Caesarian Section, at the same time.

This seemed straightforward, and I felt comfortable with the decision. Patients, in different emotional states, can decide to 'tie-off' and later regret it. Life circumstances change: couples separate, divorce and remarry, or some are widowed. Any of these could lead to a renewed desire for children, so we try to educate about these possibilities when discussing tubal ligation. During counselling, we aim to cover all these issues and more.

Both the medical team and the patient must be comfortable with the decision. We try to avoid directive counselling, although I remember a case involving a 19-year-old in her fourth pregnancy. Her mother begged me to 'tie her off'. (Oh, the family situations we find ourselves in, as physicians) Ultimately, the young woman decided to go ahead with the BTL.

In this case however, I was satisfied that we'd covered all the bases. The 38-year-old and her spouse supported the decision and encouraged it. With three children already, they felt no need for more.

Labor and delivery were normal, and we scheduled the tubal ligation for the next day. Anesthetics and the operating room were notified and prepared. The patient was being prepped, and the consent form awaited signatures. In our institution, a married spouse must also sign. When he was presented with the form and saw 'husband' specifically indicated, something shifted.

There was a pause... a silence... and then a chill entered the room. You could hear a pin drop. The eerie stillness felt like it stretched forever. The nurse and I exchanged glances and excused ourselves. We couldn't explain what had happened or understand what was going on, even after stepping out to commiserate. This sudden shift was unlike anything we'd witnessed, especially for the senior nurse in the room.

But I had a responsibility. If the procedure was to happen, the consent form had to be signed. I couldn't keep the operating room staff waiting indefinitely; the case was either on or off. Gathering my courage, I went back in to address them and decide on our next steps. With the tension slightly reduced, he asked to be excused and left. She asked to speak to me privately.

She was entirely confused. No one had explained that someone else would need to sign the consent form. She'd assumed that whether or not she wanted more children was entirely her decision. While she appreciated that her spouse of fourteen years was involved, it was her call.

I listened carefully, and that's when "the penny dropped."

Although she and her spouse had built a stable life and home with their three children, she was still legally married to someone else. Her 'husband' had his own stable household. Though they hadn't formally communicated, there was no animosity. I was floored - lost and bewildered.

I'd found myself in an incredibly embarrassing situation. It hadn't crossed my mind that she wasn't married to her current spouse; his name appeared as her next of kin on all registration forms, both in our office and at the hospital. They were a stable, supportive family. I had no reason to suspect otherwise.

All this confusion fell on my shoulders, and I had to take responsibility for the embarrassment it caused. I felt a little stupid and ashamed, replaying all those early lessons in medical school - about taking thorough histories... especially social and family history. This was her second pregnancy with me as her obstetrician, which only made my oversight more painful.

What a colossal mess I'd caused. This conversation was confidential; I couldn't rush out and tell the nurse what I'd just learned. The only help I had was a quick prayer for divine guidance. I was hoping for a pity party that wasn't coming anytime soon, so I waited for an angel to fly in. What an awful feeling.

A ray of light did shine through. Without revealing any confidential information, I informed my colleagues and the OR staff that the couple needed more time to consider the procedure, which was entirely reasonable. This pause could reduce the risk of postpartum blues and future regret. She went home on the second postpartum day and scheduled a follow-up with me in two weeks.

I sought legal advice on the situation. Legally, as long as she was still married, her husband's consent was required for the procedure. By her next appointment, I was ready to advise her. Fortunately, she'd already reached out to him. Neither she nor he had considered the potential consequences for their families, if either developed a serious illness. He had no objection to signing the form and we completed the tubal ligation at her six-week follow-up.

Later, she told me that everyone involved learned from the experience. She and her husband agreed amicably to divorce, and she would soon marry her partner.

I never discussed her details with colleagues; the case remained confidential. Years later, I referenced this scenario in another clinical setting with a separated woman adamant that "it's my body, my choice" regarding her tubal ligation. She ended up travelling to a jurisdiction with different laws to have the procedure done... Legally, I could not help her, so she did what she needed to do in her mind, without any discussion with her former husband.

As I get older, I see more and more wisdom in recognizing that life is filled with shades of grey, not just black and white. Wisdom, wherever it originates, is beyond our finite minds to fully grasp. The Man from Galilee helps me decipher life's trials in ways my limited understanding cannot...

"Faith, as the Sage calls it, is a mystery I continue to explore."

The depth of despair I felt in that room, in that moment of embarrassment, was lessened only by a prayer for divine intervention. I believe I was helped and was able to move forward.

"The ultimate measure of a person is not where they stand in moments of comfort, but in times of challenge and controversy." (Proverbs 24:10)

"Cure sometimes, treat often, comfort always."
Hippocrates

COME QUICK!

It was during one of my most challenging cases early in my career that I truly understood the importance of faith in my medical practice. At the time, I was the only practicing Obstetrician-Gynaencologist in the country, serving a population of about thirty thousand - all before the advent of cellular technology.

Our emergency room was staffed by a nurse who would call the doctor as needed... but contacting the physician could be difficult, depending on their location. On this particular day, the nurse's message was terse: "Come quickly!" The patient's vital signs were unstable, and she was gasping for breath. With no time for further details, the nurse had already summoned the supervisor on duty.

I rushed to the emergency room, leaving my personal tasks unfinished. The journey took about 10-15 minutes and without any sirens to clear traffic. It felt interminable. I prayed out of necessity, not conviction.

Hoping I would arrive in time to save a life. There was no way to communicate with the nurse during my journey, and with no one else available, the trip seemed endless.

Arriving at the ER, my palms were sweaty. I remember passing a younger gentleman outside who appeared extremely worried. Our eyes met briefly, and in those few moments, so much was conveyed without words. It was later revealed that he was the patient's spouse.

Inside the room, the nurses were frantic, setting up for the emergency. I joined them quickly, establishing an intravenous line - a 'lifeline' - and took charge of the situation.

We were in a crisis. The patient was pale, her abdomen grossly distended, in obvious pain, and struggling to breathe. She was receiving oxygen through a face mask, and each breath seemed like it might be her last. It was nearly impossible to obtain a history from her due to her distress, but we determined she was pregnant.

Confirming a diagnosis required accessing the medical laboratory, which was down the hallway. The technologist had to be called in. The patient most likely needed a blood transfusion, but our "walking blood bank" system, which relied on available donors, had inherent time constraints due to limited blood storage facilities.

Further complicating the situation was the absence of ultrasound equipment and other advanced imaging studies. Our training in clinical assessment had prepared us for making decisions based solely on clinical skills, and I was confident that the patient was bleeding internally and needed to be rushed to the operating room.

Having made the decision to operate, I assembled the operating room staff. Thankfully, it was a weekend, so staff, though limited, were available to expedite the process. However, preparing for surgery still took precious time, and the situation remained dire.

As we awaited preparations, the patient's vital signs continued to deteriorate. Prayer came spontaneously, as there was little else to do but prepare for surgery. I paced the floor, praying despite not knowing exactly what to say. It was terrifying to see someone's life slipping away before my eyes. I vividly recall the flood of emotions and felt immense relief when the surgery finally began. Her abdomen was distended and seemed ready to burst.

By the time we started the operation, the patient was clinically unstable, and we still hadn't obtained blood for transfusion. Blood poured from her abdomen as if from a burst pipe, flooding the operating field. We scrambled to identify the source of the bleeding and eventually located active bleeding from one of the fallopian tubes. The blood was pale and almost watery.

We managed to stop the bleeding, but by then the patient had almost completely exsanguinated. Despite our best efforts, she sadly expired in the operating room. This was my first experience as the lead physician in our community hospital facing such a traumatic situation.

The range of human emotions was overwhelming: guilt, sadness, anxiety and pure despair. The hardest part was facing the spouse (who was anxiously waiting outside). Having to tell him his wife had passed away was especially difficult – but ultimately this was part of the job I signed up for so long ago.... Then to leave his side and return to comfort the staff who were also distraught - it was a very difficult day.

Our collective grief left little room for Faith on that day. But once back in my car, while driving home, I began to open my mind and asked God for help in our healing - knowing that somewhere, someday, we would understand why this madness happened to such a lovely family.

"If you fall to pieces in a crisis, there wasn't
much to you in the first place."
Proverbs 24:10

JOURNAL 19

WAITING FOR DIVINE HELP

"The only thing we have to fear is fear itself."

These words, spoken by former U.S. President Franklin D. Roosevelt in 1933, echoed in my mind as I faced one of the greatest challenges of my medical career. It was the middle of the night in the operating room and the patient's bleeding was uncontrollable. She had developed the rare bleeding disorder known as Disseminated Intravascular Coagulation (DIC) - one of the most feared complications of blood clotting in obstetrics.

It was around 2 a.m., and we had been in the OR for nearly two hours with no resolution in sight. We were at our wits' end. Earlier that night, the patient began experiencing severe abdominal pain. They were constant, unrelenting and distinct from the typical pain of labor. Her abdomen was rock-hard. We quickly recognized that she had developed abruptio placentae - the separation of the placenta from the uterus - a true obstetric emergency requiring an immediate Caesarean section. She was prepped, all protocols were followed, and we took her to the OR.

While repairing the uterus, we encountered some difficulties - nothing particularly alarming at first. We retraced our steps and performed the necessary actions, but soon noticed an insidious oozing of blood at the incision site. At first, it didn't seem extraordinary. We applied standard procedures to stop the bleeding and waited. As we waited, fatigue began to set in because by now, it was past midnight, and we were all exhausted. It had been a full day already, and we all secretly longed to go home.

As the hours passed, the constant oozing persisted, raising alarms. The need for a blood transfusion became inevitable, but obtaining blood at such an hour was an arduous task in our small community hospital. The room grew increasingly tense as the specter of DIC loomed, and the realization of its possibility became undeniable. Fear gripped us. This was a midnight cry, and the atmosphere was heavy with dread.

Despite our efforts, the bleeding continued, and obtaining blood was still hours away. The potential outcome of DIC hung over us - a grim prospect that often proves fatal. My assistant was visibly fatigued, and weariness became our collective companion.

When the situation worsened, we made the dreadful decision to perform an emergency Caesarean hysterectomy - the removal of the uterus. It was now a do-or-die scenario; the alternative was losing the patient on the operating table.

Fear, fatigue, and fright shadowed us as we faced the reality of being in the OR for another two to three hours. Despite everything, we pressed on, buoyed by prayer, which had become our steadfast companion. Summoning every ounce of energy and courage, we performed the hysterectomy.

In the midst of this ordeal, a glimmer of hope appeared: two units of fresh blood arrived for transfusion. It felt as though an angel had descended from the heavens, lifting some of the weight from our weary souls. This small miracle answered a desperate prayer and brought much-needed relief.

After completing the hysterectomy, another positive sign emerged: the bleeding began to subside. By this time, we had been in the OR for over five hours. It was now early morning, and we were all on the verge of total exhaustion. Every encouraging sign felt like an answer to prayer - as if God knew we had reached the limits of human endurance.

As the team leader, I had to project optimism despite the fear and nerve-wracking experience. I can't claim my faith was particularly strong during those hours - I was a wreck. Yet I prayed continually because I simply had no other option. I can't confidently say it was my prayers that made the difference. What I do know is that there was little else to rely on in those grueling moments.

"If faith must be tested, then this was faith in action."

To suggest that we succeeded purely because of my faith would be a stretch. Fear was my constant companion as well, and I prayed against it. The mystery of faith and how God answers prayers remains a daily struggle for me. By grace, I believe, we all pressed on.

Our shift left the hospital that morning around 8 a.m., with the sun shining brightly, holding onto a fragile hope that everything would turn out all right. We were utterly spent - physically, mentally, and emotionally. The patient was still not out of danger, and the situation remained precarious. But we left knowing we had done all we could, as the new shift of nurses took over to give the patient new energy, they also gave us, the surgical team, the well-needed rest we deserved.

Later that day, I returned to the hospital. After careful consideration, we decided to transfer the patient overseas for more intensive management. We simply did not have the resources to handle further complications. The turmoil of that night still haunts me... The fear was relentless and overwhelming! It was ever present and shook us to the core.

In my readings, I've learned that faith doesn't earn us anything; rather, it draws us closer to God and gives Him opportunities to work on our behalf. The challenges of daily life create their own trials, which I try not to confuse with the trials of faith. I'm not sure how successful I am in this regard. But what I do know is how crippling fear can be. Combined with exhaustion, as it was in this case, it brought us to our knees.

Somehow, I believe my prayers - though childlike and desperate, truly made a difference. I wish I could articulate it better, but words fail me. That night, it felt as though the patient's life-changing experience rippled through all of us, leaving an indelible mark. Together, we faced the brink of life and death. In the end, not only did she survive, but we as a team were forever changed.

During difficult times like this, it's easy to let fear rule your heart. But in positions of responsibility, you must find the strength to press on. Trusting and believing, as I've learned, lies in the unseen hand of the Almighty. Though I don't physically see Him, I sense His presence. Perhaps Anne Frank said it best:

"He who has courage and faith will never perish in misery."

"If you are able, all things can be done for those who believes."
Mark 9:23

JOURNAL 20

UNCERTAINTY

Some of the most profound lessons in my medical career came not from the classroom, but from the quiet whispers of faith during moments of uncertainty. The times when I wished that help would walk through the operating room door - but it didn't. The moments when I would say to myself in the most desperate of ways, "Oh Dear God! No, not now... Why me? Why this? Why now?" These misgivings and doubts seemed to enter my soul even more during times when I'd have to perform a surgical procedure not exactly in my area of expertise.

I did have a colleague - Dr. D. O. Smith. He was also a surgeon, and we worked alongside each other daily for a period of nine years. It was just the two of us in our community hospital with surgical expertise, except for the occasional visiting surgeon. We had grown to deeply appreciate each other's help and support, but there were times when one of us was travelling, and the other was left to run the OR alone. I became acutely aware that there was no backup on the island when he travelled, and I'd be on my own.

The truth of the matter was, I needed Dr. Smith more than he needed me. I prayed regularly when he was off-island, that there would be no major incidents... but inevitably, there often were. And in retrospect, some of these were mind-boggling! Although I have struggled with the mystery of faith, and my own faith in particular - I found it to be my only reliable constant companion, especially when I was alone.

A great example of this was when I had scheduled on my regular surgery list a patient's myomectomy (removal of fibroids)... but suddenly, my colleague had to travel on emergency business. I considered postponing the surgery, but this was difficult, given both his travels and the patient's needs. However, I was confident I could proceed with the nurse's assistance, and so I did.

The senior nurse assisting me was no neophyte. We had successfully performed many cesarean sections together and I didn't expect any complications.

Knowing that I didn't have the usual assistance from Dr. Smith, I made all the necessary adjustments, including a prayer for guidance. I took the necessary precautions, understanding that this is a surgery notorious for excessive blood loss if the procedure is prolonged - so the extra measures were in place, and together my team and I proceeded.

Everything progressed smoothly initially, and we were about three-quarters of the way through the surgery when, all of a sudden, we experienced an unexpected complication...

To my surprise, I panicked. Fortunately for the rest of the staff, my panic was internal. I had a mental block... I knew I was missing something - but what? I paused, took a deep breath, and stared toward the entrance of the operating theatre as if someone had just walked in. It was a subconscious moment, hoping that Dr. Smith had miraculously arrived at the appointed time.

Being accustomed to having a colleague assisting in surgery provides confidence and reassurance. The assistant often recognizes something the lead surgeon doesn't and points it out - it's teamwork. That sort of support is invaluable and is easily missed when it is not available.

This was one of those instances when I wished my colleague were there. He most likely would have seen the roadblock and prevented the complication. The jolt I felt made me acutely aware of his absence, and my anxiety intensified momentarily. I had to inhale deeply and wake myself from the slumber of this dread confronting me. It was becoming apparent that no one was coming through that door... I cursed at myself for the sick feeling growing inside. I began to beat myself up that I had even proceeded with this surgery... I should have known better.

There was however, a corollary to this. I began to imagine that perhaps someone had walked through the operating room door. And I started to bargain with Him. I thought it best to make a deal with God: "If You help me out of my tribulation, I'll be so good! I will do Your Will."

There seemed to be no reply, and soon I felt a deep sense of longing in my plea. "What a pathetic state I'm in with this woman's life on the life!" I said to myself... but reality soon took hold of me, and I quickly reminded myself of where I was, and that I needed to stop looking for help from another. I just needed to get back to the matter at hand.

I then reflected on my old friend, Mr. Cline. He reminded me to pray daily, but especially during times of need, such as this. So, with my hands still covered in the patient's blood, I closed my eyes and whispered a quiet, earnest prayer. Seconds later, a peaceful calm entered my spirit. I sighed, thanked God, and proceeded through the difficulties with God's Unseen Hand guiding me the rest of the way. That mental block I had, was soon gone...

It is interesting to me that during those moments of desperation, the air is filled with such seriousness. But over time, humor enters into the memory of it, as if to lighten the load.

Fast forward two years later, I was at a medical conference, where I was a keynote speaker and presented my talk titled, "Myomectomy in a Small Community Hospital." I shared this experience as part of the presentation. Only this time, I found myself using a lot of medical humor while telling the story. As the audience erupted into laughter, it became apparent that every surgeon in attendance could relate to this feeling of utter desperation while having a mental block. Humor was by default, our reliable friend to help us cope with such stressful situations. We've all had moments of uncertainty, and I believe in the end, that humor (along with faith and optimism) becomes our soothing friend.

At the end of the conference, a senior doctor from the Bahamas (whom I highly respected for his reputation through a colleague) approached me with enthusiasm. He greeted me warmly and gave me a big hug. He said the most encouraging words, "Keep that humor in your work and future presentations. Well done!"

As I thanked him, his kind words struck me, and suddenly I had an 'ah-ha' moment. I realised that subconsciously, I had infused humor into my talk as a coping mechanism... not only for myself, but for everyone else in the room.

This was a great reminder that in times of darkness, we need to infuse humor and lighten up. It was during this brief conversation that I discovered the senior doctor had already learned this valuable lesson of keeping the spirit bright through laughter, long ago. It was a lesson I hold onto dearly and have used ever since as inspiration during trying times.

In my more recent working experiences with a mature and retrospective point of view, I reflect on moments like these. Having to support and encourage my younger colleagues, I often share stories like this and reassure them of the importance of faith in their own lives. We all need each other, and while our work may be different, I remind them that there will be times of difficulty when a helping hand is not readily accessible.

But faith will be…

I remind them of the words of the Muslim Scholar, Ibn Taymiyyah:

"Don't depend too much on anyone in this world, because even your own shadow leaves you when you are in the dark."

ABOUT THE AUTHOR

Dr. Kedrick Pickering: A Visionary Leader and
Dedicated Physician
Written Nov. 29, 2024

Dr. Kedrick Pickering (born April 8, 1958) is a celebrated
physician, public servant and environmental advocate
whose life's work has been dedicated to the advancement
and well-being of the Virgin Islands, also known as the
British Virgin Islands (BVI).

As a former Deputy Premier and Minister of Natural
Resources and Labour, Dr. Pickering has left an indelible
mark on the territory, driving initiatives in sustainable
development, environmental conservation, and
infrastructure growth, including the expansion of the
BVI's airport. Balancing a thriving medical career with
his commitment to public service, Dr. Pickering
continues to embody the values of leadership, dedication,
and community spirit.

Born and raised in the vibrant community of Long Look,
East End, Tortola, Dr Pickering's story is deeply
intertwined with the history and resilience of his family.
His father, an orphan born in Cuba, was adopted by
Alvin Pickering, a Virgin Islander who instilled in him the
values of perseverance, integrity, and community. These
principles shaped the foundation of Dr Pickering's life
and remain at the core of his professional and personal
endeavours.

His educational journey began at the BVI High School (now Elmore Stout High School) and continued at the University of the West Indies, where he earned his Bachelor of Medicine, Bachelor of Surgery, and Doctor of Medicine degrees. He later became a Fellow of the American College of Obstetrics and Gynaecology (FACOG), based in Washington, D.C., solidifying his standing as a highly regarded physician.

Dr. Pickering's medical career is distinguished by his service in both public health and private practice. As a government consultant Obstetrician/Gynaecologist, he played a pivotal role in improving healthcare access in the territory. Today, he continues to maintain a private practice and co-owns a multi-service medical centre, reflecting his lifelong commitment to the health and well-being of his community.

Entering public office in 1999, Dr. Pickering quickly earned a reputation as a dedicated and effective leader. Over four terms, he gained overwhelming support, securing up to 70% of the vote in his district. As Deputy Premier from 2011 to 2019, he spearheaded transformative initiatives, including the Caribbean Challenge Initiative to protect marine and coastal resources, chairing the European Union-Overseas Countries and Territories Forum, and shaping the BVI's Climate Change Policy. His work in natural resource management highlighted his deep commitment to sustainability and the preservation of the islands' natural beauty.

A passionate advocate for youth and sports, Dr. Pickering's early years as an athlete and coach reflect his dedication to fostering resilience and teamwork within his community.

These experiences, along with his father's, inspired his ongoing efforts to uplift others through education, healthcare, and public service.

Married to Alice Marie Pickering in 1993, and a proud father of four, Dr. Kedrick Pickering continues to reside in the community where his journey began... Through his enduring contributions to medicine, governance and environmental advocacy, he honors the legacy of his parents and grandparents and serves as a beacon of hope, progress and compassion for the Virgin Islands and beyond

What Fellows Are Saying About this Book:

"Powerful and inspiring, but even more thrilling to see a testament of how faith and medicine intersect and the peace that can come from allowing that intersection. Medicine is the one profession that allows us to experience the awesomeness of the Creator because we are indeed 'fearfully and wonderfully made.' Practicing from that perspective makes the practice a calling and not simply a profession! This promises to be a great read, and I'm looking forward to it! Congratulations!" – Dr June M. Samuel - the Interim Chief Executive Officer and Chief of Medical Staff at the BVI Health Services Authority (BVIHSA)

"The introduction to your book is wonderful and I can hear your voice as I read it! Thanks for sharing…. I have great anticipation for the book's publication! Blessings" - Jack Willome

"Kedrick, this is an excellent introduction. I can't wait to get a chance to purchase the final publication. I am so thankful you have taken the time to capture your thoughts of how God has moved through your life as you cared for others. You are a good friend. " - Timothy Lynn Burchfield, Consul General Guatemala

HOW TO CONTACT KEDRICK

Dr. Kedrick Pickering is also a Motivational Speaker...

If you've enjoyed this book, consider bringing Dr. Kedrick Pickering's Inspirational Message to Your Event!

Are you, or an associate, looking for a dynamic and transformative speaker to inspire, educate, and motivate your audience? Kedrick's powerful insights, engaging storytelling, and practical wisdom from his journeys of walking in faith - captivate audiences and leave a lasting impact.

Why Choose Dr Kedrick?

- **Expertise:** With years of experience as an Emergency Room Surgeon, Physician, Obstetrician/Gynecologist, and Member of the House of Representatives - Dr. Pickering has lived daily in stressful, life-and-death situations and offers actionable strategies to release fear, overcome challenges and unlock potential.

- **Engaging Presence:** Kedrick's ability to connect with audiences of all backgrounds ensures an engaging and memorable experience.

- **Tailored Topics:** From personal development to walking in faith, Kedrick's presentations are customizable to meet the needs of your audience.

Book Kedrick Today!

Whether it's a corporate event, conference, or workshop, Kedrick's inspiring presentations are always in demand... To inquire on Dr. Pickering's availability for your next event, please visit:

www.KedrickPickering.com

or email:

info@KedrickPickering.com

Signature Speaking Topics:

- "Leadership in Healing: What Every Professional Can Learn from Serving a Community in Need"
- "The Interconnection of Women's Health & Relationships"
- "The Menopausal & Post-Menopausal Woman - What Everyone Should Know"
- "Bridging Science and Spirituality: A Doctor's Walk with Faith and Healing"
- "Faith, Focus, and Leadership: Timeless Lessons for Today's Business and Community Leaders"
- "Service Beyond Borders: Lessons in Humanity from an Island Surgeon"

Talks range from 10 minutes to 3 hours in length.

Contact to discuss possibilities
  info@kedrickpickering.com

We look forward to sharing more about Dr. Kedrick Pickering's speaking availability, and how he can bring value to your next corporate conference or event.

Notes & Thoughts:

Walk In Faith & Medicine

.

www.ingramcontent.com/pod-product-compliance
Lightning Source LLC
Chambersburg PA
CBHW061650120626
46550CB00003B/889